'*What do I need to do to make a difference?* might be our most important and frequently asked question as clinicians. In this insightful and accessible presentation of Clinical Cases in Dysarthria, well-known authors and editors Margaret Walshe and Nick Miller describe, together with invited authors, a number of relevant and informative case examples, cases that reveal the depth and complexity of the communication problems faced by individuals with dysarthria and their clinicians. And they do it with the passion to make a difference. Walshe and Miller provide us with an opportunity to learn from individuals and to thereby find principles to apply in other cases. We gain new perspectives, rather than just solving problems'.

Professor Lena Hartelius, *Department of Health and Rehabilitation, University of Gothenburg, Sweden*

There are a multitude of valuable ways to study and improve the evaluation, diagnosis and care of people with dysarthria. The cases in this book illustrate more effectively than any randomized controlled trial or rigorously-controlled single-subject study that optimal real-world clinical care for people with dysarthria is an art based on science. This book exemplifies the great educational and heuristic value of case studies from expert clinicians and experienced researchers who understand the importance of evidence in diagnostic and treatment decision-making, while maintaining a central focus on the needs of our patients within the world in which they live.

Professor Joseph R. Duffy, *Emeritus Consultant & Professor Speech Pathology, Mayo Clinic, Rochester, USA*

T0373645

Clinical Cases in Dysarthria

Through the medium of detailed clinical case reports, written by well-respected clinicians and researchers working internationally in the field, *Clinical Cases in Dysarthria* discusses the challenges, and rewards of applying evidence-based procedures to people with dysarthria in real-life busy routine clinical settings.

The text opens with an introduction to the latest research and practices within dysarthria treatment and sets the scene for the eight individual case reports which follow. These case reports form the core chapters of the text and cover themes that range from clinical diagnostic conundrums to applying popular, and/or novel intervention approaches to different populations where dysarthria presents. Each chapter has a specific argument drawing on theoretical principles of assessment and rehabilitation, incorporating latest research evidence to help readers problem-solve similar cases in their clinical practice. Throughout the text, readers are encouraged to 'think outside the box'.

This book will be essential for undergraduate and postgraduate student clinicians within speech and language therapy/pathology courses, as well as clinicians new to the field of dysarthria.

Margaret Walshe is Associate Professor in Trinity College Dublin, Ireland. She is also a speech and language therapist with extensive experience in dysarthria and related disorders. Her current research is focused on the amalgamation of evidence for intervention approaches in speech and swallowing disorders associated with acquired neurodegenerative disease.

Nick Miller is Emeritus Professor of Motor Speech Disorders at the University of Newcastle, UK. His internationally acclaimed research has been based on single case and small group studies through to large-scale investigatory and experimental approaches, qualitative as well as quantitative methods. He continues to be an active researcher, with particular emphasis on apraxia of speech, dysarthria and functional/psychogenic speech disorders.

Clinical Cases in Speech and Language Disorders

Clinical Cases in Speech and Language Disorders is a new series of short books that each focus on a specific speech and language disorder, providing an in-depth look at real or imagined scenarios, and discussing relevant assessment and intervention plans using theory, research findings, and clinical reasoning. The overall aim of these books is to provide much-needed resources using real-life clinical cases to help clinicians and students reflect on clinical decision making involving the assessment and management of patients presenting with various speech and language disorders (SLD).

Titles in the series

Clinical Cases in Dysarthria
Edited by Margaret Walshe and Nick Miller

Clinical Cases in Dysphagia
Edited by Margaret Walshe and Maggie-Lee Huckabee

For more information about this series, please visit: www.routledge.com/Clinical-Cases-in-Speech-and-Language-Disorders/book-series/CCSLD

Clinical Cases in Dysarthria

Edited by Margaret Walshe and Nick Miller

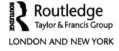

Routledge
Taylor & Francis Group

LONDON AND NEW YORK

First published 2022
by Routledge
2 Park Square, Milton Park, Abingdon, Oxon OX14 4RN

and by Routledge
605 Third Avenue, New York, NY 10158

Routledge is an imprint of the Taylor & Francis Group, an informa business

British Library Cataloguing-in-Publication Data
A catalogue record for this book is available from the British Library

Library of Congress Cataloging-in-Publication Data
Names: Walshe, Margaret, editor. | Miller, Nick, editor.
Title: Clinical cases in dysarthria/edited by Margaret Walshe, Nick Miller.
Description: Milton Park, Abingdon, Oxon; New York, NY: Routledge, 2022.
Series: Clinical cases in speech and language disorders | Includes bibliographical references and index.
Identifiers: LCCN 2021031607 (print) | LCCN 2021031608 (ebook) | ISBN 9781032000572 (hardback) | ISBN 9781032000565 (paperback) | ISBN 9781003172536 (ebook)
Subjects: LCSH: Articulation disorders—Case studies.
Classification: LCC RC424.7.C55 2022 (print) | LCC RC424.7 (ebook) | DDC 616.85/5—dc23
LC record available at https://lccn.loc.gov/2021031607
LC ebook record available at https://lccn.loc.gov/2021031608

ISBN: 978-1-032-00057-2 (hbk)
ISBN: 978-1-032-00056-5 (pbk)
ISBN: 978-1-003-17253-6 (ebk)

DOI: 10.4324/9781003172536

Typeset in Garamond
by Apex CoVantage, LLC

Access the Support Materials: www.routledge.com/9781032000565

We dedicate this book to people living with dysarthria and to the clinicians who work tirelessly to make a difference to their lives.

Contents

Figures and tables

Tables

Figures

Contributors

Irene Battel, PhD, is a senior speech and language therapist at the Ospedale Civile di Venezia Santi Giovanni e Paolo, Venice, Italy. Her clinical specialisms include management of complex dysphagia and dysarthria in a neurological and neuromuscular population as well as critical care in the intensive care unit. As Italy became the first western country to experience the coronavirus disease 2019 (COVID-19) epidemic, she was involved early in the management of people with COVID-19. She currently teaches at the University of Padova, Italy. Her research interests are neurogenic dysphagia and implementation of principles of motor learning in dysphagia and speech rehabilitation programmes.

Suzanne Beeke, PhD, is Associate Professor at University College London, GB. She trained as a speech and language therapist, and her research is focused on understanding the impact of language and communication disorders on the everyday conversations of adults with acquired neurological conditions. She is a lead author of Better Conversations with Aphasia, a free online training resource and therapy programme available at https://extendstore.ucl.ac.uk

Jennifer Benson, M.Sc., is a speech and language therapist, with over 20 years' experience in adult neurology. She has a particular interest and specialism in motor neurone disease (MND). This led to her establishing the first service in the United Kingdom to offer voice banking to all newly diagnosed patients with MND. She has presented both nationally and internationally on this topic and continues to be committed to promoting its benefits to people with MND and other conditions.

Steven Bloch, PhD, is Associate Professor and Head of the Clinical Speech and Language Sciences Programme at University College London. GB. He has 30 years' clinical and research experience in working with people with acquired progressive neurological conditions. His research interests include the application of conversation analytical methods to the study of dysarthria, augmentative and alternative communication use and end-of-life care.

Elizabeth Cardell, PhD, is Professor of Speech Pathology at Griffith University, Queensland, Australia. She had a long clinical career in neurological rehabilitation prior to entering full-time academia and has published widely in the area of acquired neurogenic communication and swallowing disorders. She has pioneered new treatment and service delivery models for the management of aphasia, dysarthria and swallowing and has a particular interest in neuroplasticity and the principles of motor learning and how these can be translated to day-to-day practice optimising treatment outcomes.

Emma Finch, PhD, is a conjoint senior research fellow between the University of Queensland and the Princess Alexandra Hospital, Brisbane, Australia. Her key research areas are improving participation following acquired communication disorders and research capacity building.

Annie Hill, PhD, is a senior postdoctoral researcher with the Centre for Research Excellence in Aphasia Recovery and Rehabilitation and a founding member of the Centre for Research in Telerehabilitation at the School of Health and Rehabilitation Sciences, the University of Queensland, Australia. Annie's research programme is focused on clinical assessment and treatment of acquired swallowing and communication disorders in adults, and her research has led to impacts in health service re-design and end-user engagement in technology codesign.

Leslie Mahler, PhD, CCC-SLP, MBA, is Professor in the Department of Communicative Disorders at the University of Rhode Island, USA. She has over 35 years of clinical experience in evaluation, diagnosis and treatment of dysarthria. She worked as a speech-language pathologist in a medical setting prior to earning a dual doctorate in Speech and Hearing Sciences and Neuroscience from the University of Colorado-Boulder in 2006. The main focus of her research is the integration of principles of motor learning that drive activity-dependent changes in neural plasticity to improve treatment outcomes for people with dysarthria. Dr. Mahler teaches courses in Motor Speech Disorders, Dysphagia, and Acquired Cognitive Disorders while maintaining an active clinical practice at the University of Rhode Island.

Nick Miller, PhD, FRCSLT, is Emeritus Professor of Motor Speech Disorders at the University of Newcastle, GB. His career has involved posts in clinical management of people with acquired progressive and non-progressive neurological communication disorders in community and hospital settings and latterly also lecturing and research on these and related topics. His internationally acclaimed research has been based on single case and small group studies through to large-scale investigatory and experimental approaches, qualitative as well as quantitative methods. He continues to be an active researcher, with a particular emphasis on apraxia of speech, dysarthria and functional/psychogenic speech disorders.

Stacie Park, PhD, is a speech-language pathologist with a clinical background in acute care and neurorehabilitation. She was awarded her PhD by the University of Queensland, Australia, in 2018 for her thesis which described the development of a novel intensive speech treatment for non-progressive dysarthria. Her research interests include best practice for the management of dysarthria following acquired brain injury and telerehabilitation.

Rachael Rietdijk, PhD, is a speech-language pathologist and post-doctoral research fellow in the Sydney School of Health Sciences at the University of Sydney, Australia. She completed her PhD in 2019 at the University of Sydney and focused on the use of telepractice for communication partner training after traumatic brain injury. She is currently working on a project funded by icare New South Wales, Australia, to develop *The Social Brain Toolkit*, which is a suite of online tools to support communication skills after brain injury.

Deborah Theodoros, PhD, is an emeritus professor at the University of Queensland, Brisbane, Australia. She is a speech pathologist with over 40 years of clinical and research experience. She has held a continuing teaching and research position at the University of Queensland from 1995 to 2019. She has an established programme of research across two core areas: the management of motor speech and voice disorders, involving intensive treatment protocols, and the development, validation and implementation of telepractice in speech pathology.

Margaret Walshe, PhD, is Associate Professor at Trinity College Dublin, Ireland. To date, she has supervised over 80 postgraduate research projects in speech and swallowing disorders and evidence-based practice. She is a speech and language therapist with over 30 years of clinical experience in dysarthria and related disorders. She completed her PhD in dysarthria in 2003 on the psychosocial impact of dysarthria from the speaker's perspective. Her current research is focused on the amalgamation of evidence for intervention approaches in speech and swallowing disorders associated with acquired neurodegenerative disease.

Brooke-Mai Whelan, PhD, is a lecturer in speech pathology in the School of Health and Rehabilitation Sciences at the University of Queensland, Australia. Her research interests include the efficacy of adult speech rehabilitation following acquired brain injury, neural mechanisms underpinning motor speech recovery and telerehabilitation. She led the research into the telerehabilitation delivery of the Be Clear intervention for dysarthria.

Preface

Despite being the most commonly acquired communication disorder, dysarthria seems to lag behind other areas in speech-language pathology in terms of the intensity of research into the field and consequent advances in assessment and clinical practice. Yet, becoming dysarthric can be devastating for the individual, tearing at the very heart of who one is as a person, with significant repercussions that go way beyond the individual. As two long established clinicians and researchers, we strongly believe that there is so much to offer to make a difference for people with dysarthria and their families. Our clinical research work to date reflects this conviction.

Clinical Cases in Dysarthria, part of the larger *Clinical Cases* series, provided us with an opportunity to seek out similar minded people who share that passion to make a difference in how we manage dysarthria and for people with dysarthria. The *Clinical Cases* series does not seek to provide exhaustive systematic reviews of current knowledge or a detailed recipe book of 'how to'. Rather, it aims through the medium of detailed clinical case reports to illustrate the challenges and rewards of applying evidence-based procedures to real cases in a real-life busy routine clinical setting. Case reports can be powerful in helping to understand more fully clinical presentations, clinical decision-making processes and 'thinking on one's feet'.

We hope that this can give an immediacy and relevance to appreciating and applying the evidence base in different areas that is often lacking from more theoretical treatises, especially for student clinicians or colleagues new to the field of dysarthria.

The invited authors have selected case reports from their research or clinical practice to support some key messages within their text. Most chapters are extended through the use of additional supplementary material, including videos. These will help the reader gain a deeper understanding of elements associated with the case reports within the chapters. These resources should also prove invaluable in piquing further interest and promoting clinical discussion.

The text begins with a brief overview of dysarthria assessment and management. The remaining chapters illustrate key current issues in assessment and intervention in a range of different speakers, including people with dysarthria post-traumatic brain injury, stroke, Parkinson's disease, of widely different ages, personal circumstances and reactions to dysarthria, across a variety of settings (domiciliary, hospital and telehealth).

Of course, even with this breadth of coverage, we appreciate that this (or any other single work) cannot come close to capturing the myriad facets of dysarthria, its presentation and how it affects individual speakers. Thus, there are undoubtedly unavoidable omissions. Nevertheless, we trust that this text provides a useful starting point and templates for considering evidence-based approaches in a real-life contexts for people with dysarthria.

Margaret Walshe
Nick Miller
Month 2021

Abbreviations

AAC	Alternative and augmentative communication
AIDS	The Assessment of Intelligibility of Dysarthric Speech
BC	Better conversations
BCD	Better conversations with dysarthria
CARE	CAse REports
CBT	Cognitive behavioural therapy
CER	Communication efficiency ratio
CES	Communication Effectiveness Survey
CETI-M	Communication Effectiveness Index-Modified
COVID-19	Novel coronavirus SARS-CoV-2
CP	Conversation partner
CPAP	Continuous Positive Airway Pressure
CPIB	Communication Participation Item Bank
dB	Decibels
DDK	Diadochokinesis
DIP	Dysarthria impact profile
DME	Direct magnitude estimation
DS	Down syndrome
EMG	Electromyography
FRDA	Friedreich's ataxia
FUP	Follow-up
GRBAS	Grade, Roughness, Breathiness, Asthenia, Grade Scale
HDU	High-dependency unit
ICF	International Classification of Functioning, Disability and Health
ICU	Intensive care unit
IOPI	Iowa Oral Performance Instrument
IWPM	Intelligible words per minute
KP	Knowledge of performance
kPa	Kilopascal (unit of measurement)
KR	Knowledge of results
LSVT/LSVT LOUD	Lee Silverman Voice Treatment

MAIC	Motor Accident Insurance Commission
MND	Motor neurone disease
MoCA	Montreal Cognitive Assessment
MRI	Magnetic resonance imaging
MSA	Multiple system atrophy
NG	Nasogastric tube
OME	Oro-motor examination
PaO_2	Partial pressure of oxygen
QOL-Dys	Quality of life related to dysarthria
ROM	Range of motion/movement
RCT	Randomised controlled trial
SD	Standard deviation
SLP	Speech-language pathology/pathologist
SLT	Speech and language therapy/therapist
SPL	Sound pressure levels
SVR	Surgical Voice Restoration
TBI	Traumatic brain injury
TIS	Total impact score
VSA	Vowel space area
WPM	Words per minute

Chapter 1

Dysarthria

Setting the scene

Nick Miller and Margaret Walshe

Introduction

Dysarthria denotes a neuromuscular disorder of speech. It represents probably the most prevalent speech-language disorder. It can be present from birth or be acquired at any age. Up to 53% of people after stroke may experience lasting dysarthria (Miller & Bloch, 2017); it constitutes a common long-term sequel of head injury. Dysarthria accompanies many progressive neurological disorders, with speech–voice changes reported in around 90% of people with Parkinson's disease (Miller, 2017; Miller et al., 2007; Schalling, Johansson, & Hartelius, 2017), 80% of people with motor neurone disease (Vieira, Costa, Sousa, Reis, & Coelho, 2020), 45–50% with multiple sclerosis (Noffs et al., 2018) and approaching 100% of people with multiple system atrophy and progressive supranuclear palsy (Miller, Nath, Noble, & Burn, 2017). Myasthenia gravis, Huntington's disease, Bell's palsy, Ramsay Hunt syndrome, generalised and focal dystonias, muscular dystrophies and mitochondrial disorders (Read et al., 2012) can all involve dysarthria. More than 50% of children with cerebral palsy may be impacted by dysarthria, with many experiencing difficulties into adulthood (Coleman, Weir, Ware, & Boyd, 2015; Tan et al., 2020). Dysarthric sounding speech can be a presenting symptom of functional neurological disorders (see Chapter 2).

Manifestation of dysarthria varies enormously, by cause, course, voice–speech features and severity. This chapter gives a flavour of this variety, along with implications for assessment and rehabilitation. This sets the scene for the remaining chapters, which focus on specific issues of assessment and/or intervention.

Defining dysarthria

The heart of any definition of dysarthria is that speech changes because of neurophysiological alterations to centres and pathways in the central and peripheral nervous systems that play a role in speech production. Typically, this also covers disruption from alterations at the neuromuscular junction and the electrochemistry of muscles themselves. A common account is that

DOI: 10.4324/9781003172536-1

the neuromuscular alterations alter tone, and/or power, and/or coordination of movements of the muscles for articulation, which in turn impair the force, range, rate, velocity, sustainability and differentiation of movements of speech. This tells only a fraction of the story.

One can describe dysarthric speech–voice according to changes in different subsystems (respiration, voice, resonance and articulation), sound classes (vowels–consonants, plosives, fricatives, etc.) and prosody (stress, intonation, rate and duration). This still represents a highly oversimplified sketch. The relationship between neuromuscular dysfunction and the range, rate and sustainability of movements is not straightforward. Neither is the relationship between these movement changes and intelligibility transparent (Chiu & Neel, 2020; McAuliffe, Fletcher, Kerr, O'Beirne, & Anderson, 2017; Miller, 2013). Consequently, levels of severity on instrumental clinical measures (e.g. force transducers, acoustics, and electromyography) may poorly reflect how severely communication is impacted, as experienced by the person with dysarthria and their family (see Chapter 7) (Gillivan-Murphy, Miller, & Carding, 2019; McAuliffe, Baylor, & Yorkston, 2017).

Dysarthria is not merely about not moving the articulators. Communication does not happen in a vacuum. It is a social act. Where people communicate, with whom, why and what about, makes immensely diverse demands on speech. Individuals come with a varied experience and lifetime's set of habits around speaking, as do their partners regarding how they listen to and interact with the person with dysarthria. This signals key lessons for assessing and managing dysarthria (see Chapters 7 and 9).

Equally importantly, a speaker requires vigilance and constant monitoring to maintain attention to effort to keep speech intelligible, to integrate speech with language output and to make sure the correct emotional–affective tone of voice is conveyed. Participating in conversations demands sustaining and switching attention to keep up with content; sufficient speed and capacity of processing to comprehend what is said and compose one's own responses. Conversations need appropriate non-verbal postural, facial and gestural communication to signal desire to take a turn and to maintain one's turn; ability to initiate and sustain fluent, audible speech to maintain one's turn; and so forth. All these facets may be affected in people with dysarthria. Even if someone sounds intelligible, these factors render attempts at communication cognitively and physically challenging for the speaker, again emphasising that understanding dysarthria entails far more than examination of distorted sounds.

Moreover, dysarthria exists, and assessment and rehabilitation take place, against the backdrop of diagnosis of a life-changing, possibly life-limiting condition. The individual's and family's dreams and reality have been turned upside down. They face a future of uncertainty or grim inevitability not just regarding physical, cognitive and mental health, but socially, financially and domestically too (Miller, Noble, Jones, Deane, & Gibb, 2011; Walshe & Miller, 2011; Wray & Clarke, 2017; Wray, Clarke, & Forster, 2019).

All these underline the repeatedly stressed imperative that a comprehensive, accurate characterisation of dysarthria must encompass all levels of measurement in the International Classification of Function (Hartelius & Miller, 2010). One may learn something from examining acoustic and articulatory aspects of pronunciation breakdown (impairment), but, if evaluation does not embrace activity (intelligibility and communicative ability) and psychosocial impact of dysarthria on participation in society (see Chapter 7) as well as environmental and cultural factors, one will only ever obtain a partial, distorted understanding. Without incorporating the views and roles of significant listeners in the person's environment, one sees only half the picture. Furthermore, the same profile of impairment has a different impact on intelligibility and social interaction depending on the cultural-language context of the individual. Ignoring this also diminishes one's completeness of understanding and assessment of dysarthria (Miller & Lowit, 2014).

The variety of dysarthria

Dysarthria arises in myriad ways. Dysarthria associated with cerebral palsy notwithstanding, it is mostly acquired after childhood. Onset may be sudden (e.g. stroke and head injury) or gradual (neoplasms and progressive neurological conditions).

In stroke and head injury, spontaneous improvement may occur. Resection of neoplasms may win benefits. However, the situation can be highly variable as regards whether (spontaneous) improvement happens, how long it takes or continues and whether speech ever returns to previous levels.

In degenerative conditions, progression may be rapid, gradual or stepwise, with possible periods of (partial) remission along the way. Decline can run over a few years or decades. Dysarthria may be an early severe, inevitable, relentless accompaniment to one condition, but a late occasional, mild sequel in another. For some aetiologies, alterations to voice, speech or resonance during a long prodromal period may signal the first inkling that something is amiss.

Dysarthria/dysphonia can arise as a sole manifestation of an isolated cranial nerve palsy. These cases are exceptional (see Chapter 3). Characteristically, speech alterations constitute but one element in a highly complex picture. Dysarthria exists alongside other physical (e.g. tremor, dystonia and hemiplegia), neuropsychological (e.g. aphasia and visual/auditory-perceptual dysfunction), cognitive and affective (e.g. apathy and depression) changes. Any or all of these might interact with speaking to impact on communication, complicate assessment and pose additional challenges in rehabilitation. In older people, physical, cognitive and psychosocial factors that affect communication in this age group may accompany neurological changes (Palmer et al., 2019).

The multiplicity of co-occurring conditions may colour priorities for intervention. One person is unconcerned that listeners struggle to understand what they say, their only wish is to fix their pain, disruptive dyskinesias, poor sleep, brain fog or whatever. Another person sounds as if they have nothing more than a mildly tremorous voice or hemifacial weakness scarcely impinging on speech, yet this is sufficient to cause a debilitating withdrawal from communicating (Miller, Noble, Jones, Allcock, & Burn, 2008; Walshe & Miller, 2011; Walshe, Miller, Leahy, & Murray, 2008).

Assessment

Why assess

Assessment is a *sine qua non* of evidence-based working, successful diagnosis and appropriately tailored intervention (Dobinson & Miller 2019; Lowit & Kent, 2011). It should answer why exactly the person is as they are, which factors are impacting their communication and which key elements if they can be modified will make a decisive difference to communication. Findings inform conversations between the person with dysarthria, their family and clinicians about what they want to do, where they want to be and how to get there.

What to assess

Systematic evaluation of dysarthria typically measures the pattern of performance within and across output subsystems – respiration, voice, resonance, articulation, prosody – to establish if and how any of them individually or jointly constitutes a source of reduced communicative ability.

That is a start. Since successful verbal communication is not the property of any single subsystem or articulator but emerges from interaction and coordination between all subsystems and between them and cognitive–affective variables, a vital step is to ascertain how well subsystems combine to produce viable speech/voice. For instance, respiratory support for speech may be satisfactory, but loss of air pressure due to velopharyngeal insufficiency tips the scales towards poor breath support for articulation; tongue tip to palate closure and vocal cord vibration may be independently competent, but poor timing between laryngeal and lingual subsystems leads to dysfluency or/and perceptually ambiguous voiced-voiceless realisations; lip strength may be sufficient for closure, but this is negated by inability to hold the mandible sufficiently raised. Ultimately, judging how well subsystems combine successfully comes from intelligibility evaluation (Lousada, Jesus, Hall, & Joffe, 2014; Miller, 2013; Sescleifer, Francoisse, & Lin, 2018; Wannberg, Schalling, & Hartelius, 2016).

Prosody components such as stress placement and intonation convey essential signals to listeners, not just meaning content but also emotional content. For some people with dysarthria, prosodic changes represent the chief factor undermining communication. Furthermore, a monoloud or monotone voice can contribute to negative perception of speakers. Therefore, inclusion of ability to convey differences in meaning dependent on stress and intonation and signalling different emotional content (sad, happy, tentative, etc.) is indispensable.

Because communication is a social act, assessment of the individual's communicative environment, how communication changes have impacted on them, their views on where, when, why and how they wish to communicate and the roles and views of significant listeners are as important as any narrower focus on voice, speech and gesture examination (see Chapters 7 and 9). Given the non-linear relationship between physiological impairment, intelligibility and perceived impact on participation, meaningful assessment must combine all these strands. Attention, speed of processing, language, non-verbal and gestural communication and the pragmatics of managing conversations are candidates for evaluation.

How to assess

Many major texts on motor speech disorders offer detailed directions for assessment (Duffy, 2019; Hixon, Weismer, & Holt, 2008; Lowit & Kent, 2011). Table 1.1 outlines a basic framework (see Chapter 2 for more on differential diagnosis). It does not dictate that every single test must be completed at every assessment point. What is essential is that a clinical hypothesis is formulated, regular evaluation happens, conducted in a standardised, valid and reliable fashion and that across assessment points like is compared with like, free of possible tester, listener and environmental biases.

Oral non-verbal movements are not included as their relevance in speech assessment is questionable (Kent, 2015; Maas, 2017; Mackenzie, Muir, Allen, & Jensen, 2014; Ziegler & Ackermann, 2013). Blowing the cheeks out, reaching the tongue towards the nose or pressing on a strain gauge may provide some insights into lip and tongue strength, but the results say nothing about whether the individual can produce intelligible labial and dental sounds and contrasts in speech.

Therapy/intervention

Some underlying causes of dysarthria are amenable to pharmacological or surgical interventions that slow, halt or reverse deterioration. Currently, such options remain restricted. Even then benefits may be time-limited and/or come with negative side effects, individuals need to weigh against possible advantages. The holy grail of halting, reversing or even preventing decline in the first place is the focus of widespread research. Thus, for most people with dysarthria, behavioural management by the SLT/SLP remains the main avenue to tackle their communication issues.

Table 1.1 Outline framework for assessment of communication in dysarthria

Task	Examples of valid assessments
Impairment	
Respiration/voice	Count to 20 or repeat a given syllable in time with a metronome
	Breaths required to read standard passage
	Sound pressure level metre recordings
	Jitter, shimmer, harmonics–noise ratio; mean/SD sound pressure level; laryngoscopy
	Perceptual voice rating scales
	See below 'prosody'
Resonance	Nasal spirometer; alternating oral–nasal diadochokinesis (DDK), for example, repeat 10 times 'any-eddy', 'dough-no', 'wane-wade' 'may-bay', etc.
Articulation	Diadochokinetic tasks:
	a) Time for 10 repetitions of single syllable
	b) Ability to achieve and maintain key sound contrasts across 10 repetitions – for example:
	pea-bee; pea-tea; pea-fee
	tea-see; tea-D; tea-key
	shoe-choo, too-choo; sue-shoe
	key-keep; ape-tape; loss-lost; ski-key, see-ski, will-willed
Activity	
Intelligibility	Diagnostic intelligibility test
	Minimal pair probes looking at specific sound/syllable/prosody contrasts
	Communicative success rating scales
	Listener success answering questions on standard passage content
Prosody	
Sentence/word level	Say 'no' with rising/falling intonation; 'yes' as sad, happy, tentative, angry
	DDK with varying stress/rhythm: 'paapapa vs papa'paa'; 'pa'taka vs pata'ka vs 'pata'ka
	Lexical and syntactic disambiguation: statement versus question; green 'house versus 'greenhouse; they're hunting '**dogs** versus they're '**hunting** dogs
	Mean and standard deviation of fundamental frequency on prolonged vowels and voiced phrases
Participation and impact	
Psychosocial issues	Speaker and carer questionnaires, semantic differential scales; conversational analysis

Intervention targets key variable(s) that assessment proves are significantly undermining communicative success, with methods geared to the individual's preferred manner of communication, for success in the places they wish to communicate and roles they wish to fulfil.

The diversity of ways in which dysarthria manifests and impacts on people is matched by the variety of interventions. For some, intervention addresses subtle shades of prosody in expressing emotional content of utterances, others need to commence with establishing basic vowel–vowel or consonant–vowel distinctions (he–who, he–we, who–you, etc.) or achieving optimum posture for breathing. Assessment maybe showed that slowing target speaking rate and/or raising sound pressure level significantly improves intelligibility. Equally, targets may entail key environmental modifications – creating an optimum auditory-visual space for successful communication; negotiation between partners about how best to share communicative burden; and recognising and repairing breakdowns in understanding (see Chapter 9) strategies for specific contexts – the phone, a noisy shop or a hard of hearing relative.

Intervention seldom entails single factors. Rehabilitation equips speakers with an armoury of options, combining speaker-centred work with speaker-external or collaborative strategies which are applied and adapted across time and contexts. Moreover, success in the quiet, supportive confines of a clinic room is one thing. Strategies and techniques impractical outside clinic and/or failing to incorporate into intervention appropriate methods that assure maintenance and generalisation in contexts where the skills need to be employed, means treatment will fail. Hence, the importance of methods that foster transfer and maintenance (see later), such as 'half-way house' communication groups (Whillans, Lawrie, Cardell, Kelly, & Wenke, 2020; Yorkston, Baylor, & Britton, 2017) bridging one-to-one and real-life situations, building support networks, regular homework targets even when not in active therapy (Wight & Miller, 2015), planned regular top-up sessions and apps that provide 'in the wild' real-time feedback on key speech–voice parameters (Gustafsson, Södersten, Ternström, & Schalling, 2019).

In many progressive conditions, no amount of well-principled SLT/SLP therapy can halt the inexorable march of underlying neurodegeneration. This dictates constantly balancing maximisation of what is currently possible against what will be feasible as attention, motivation, energy, motor and cognitive capability reach critical thresholds of decline. This demands a palliative and anticipatory approach from the start, with vital conversations for all concerned (Chapter 8).

Discussion may involve how to reconcile dream wishes with what is physically and cognitively feasible; negotiating a tolerable balance between independence and dependence; choices of spoken versus written, signed or alternative and augmentative communication (AAC); strategies to achieve the best in current circumstances, but simultaneously awareness of adjustments likely to happen down the line and what other factors may emerge as priorities for support. One must anticipate how to manage provision as one moves from cognitively and physically able to where status challenges ability to actively participate in therapy and communication (see Chapters 8 and 9).

Speech intervention

Handed-down wisdom suggests the order of priority when focusing narrowly on speech follows the logic of how speech is produced: commence with respiration (without air to drive the whole system, there is silence), then phonation (with no sound source there is no or only a distorted vocal note for articulators to modify) and then resonance (especially in cases where nasal escape of air/ hypernasality subvert function in other subsystems). Only with viable performance in these does one move to articulation and prosody. Older textbooks detailed many therapies directed at subsystems and neuromuscular changes underlying specific problems. Techniques such as yawn-sigh, humming, pushing and pulling to influence laryngeal tone, methods to address oral versus nasal airflow, tongue movement range, poor lip seal and so forth were advocated.

In selected instances, some of these methods may be wholly appropriate, especially if the technique is but one component of a multipronged intervention. However, there is a paucity of studies demonstrating the efficacy of most such approaches (Finch, Rumbach, & Park, 2020; Mitchell, Bowen, Tyson, Butterfint, & Conroy, 2017; Munoz-Vigueras et al., 2020; Whillans et al., 2020). Furthermore, the integrated nature of speech motor control across multiple subsystems means many have potentially serious disadvantages. Quite apart from disregarding the collaborative, psychosocial dimensions of communication, they downplay or ignore the integrated nature of speech production and adjustments to impairment that take place across multiple subsystems; they risk falling at the hurdle of incorporating gains from isolated articulators into speech control in general.

This suggests a more holistic and integrated approach. Accumulating randomised controlled trial and other strong evidence supports the efficacy of integrated strategies, demonstrating one can improve intelligibility by effecting change across multiple speech subsystems without recourse to tackling them one at a time. Amongst favoured methods are therapies targeting attention to effort (Park, Theodoros, Finch, & Cardell, 2016; Pennington, Miller, Robson, & Steen, 2010; Sackley et al., 2020; Yuan et al., 2020) (see too Chapters 4, 5 and 6) and rate manipulation (Ballard et al., 2015; Kuschmann, Miller, Lowit, & Pennington, 2017; Patel, Connaghan, & Campellone, 2013). Other significant works in recent years have also advanced our understanding of delivery of support in domiciliary settings, via telehealth (Ballard et al., 2015; Wray & Clarke, 2017; Yorkston, Baylor, & Britton, 2017) (see also Chapters 3, 5 and 6).

There is no room to review interventions in detail here. Later chapters in this text focus on many of the important methods and evidence base in specific fields. National and international advocacy organisations for different neurological conditions also provide invaluable information for professionals and affected families on communication.

Motor learning

Aside from issues above of how to manipulate voice–speech parameters, there are further factors that guide intervention, whatever the specific approach. Motor learning is one of these factors. This refers to the (re)acquisition, maintenance and generalisation of motor skills – typing, manipulating a joystick, dancing, skiing, playing the cello, pronunciation or whatever.

There has been debate concerning whether principles of motor learning established in sport and skill acquisition fields apply to speech (Kent, 2004; Kent, 2015; Maas, 2017; Schmidt, Lee, Winstein, Wulf, & Zelaznik, 2018; Shumway-Cook & Woollacott, 2016; Ziegler & Ackermann, 2013). The following looks briefly at some of the claims and arguments. The reader is directed also to Chapters 3, 4, 5 and 6.

A little practice often through the day and week is better than large chunks of infrequent practice – particularly where fatigue and fading attention are barriers. Progress demands many, many repetitions of tokens over long periods to (re)establish a skill as second nature, able to run whilst detracting as little attention from other tasks as possible. In general, progression is from simple to complex tasks/targets and from what is just about possible to what is not yet possible, all the time building on preserved skills. Goals stretch but do not overstretch. Commonly, practice moves from observation (watch/listen to me, this is what we're aiming for), to practice in unison (let's do this together), to delayed repetition after the clinician, still dependent on external feedback; thence to fading therapist support, increasing independence from clinician/device feedback and finally reliance on own monitoring and internally guided adjustments to reach target behaviours.

In terms of not relapsing to baseline once active therapy ceases and generalising learning to novel tasks, general principles argue that random practice (a bit of this, a bit of that; contrasting labial plosives with fricatives, then alveolar plosives versus fricatives; mixing old learning with new) wins out over blocked practice (concentrate exclusively on one target, only move to next when target values reached). Practising targets in a variable fashion (e.g. loud, soft, fast slow, in a variety of syllables and word positions and modes of elicitation) wins out over invariable practice (target practised every time in exactly the same way and context).

Some important provisos have arisen when transferring these principles to people with motor speech disorders. For people with dysarthria and indeed apraxia of speech (Miller & Wambaugh, 2021), even apparently simple tasks are already complex. Thus, rather than commencing directly with random, variable practice with fading, irregular feedback, a period of blocked, invariable learning may be required to get people onto the bottom rung of the skill ladder, using frequent, regular feedback.

Important contrasts between limb skill acquisition in healthy subjects and voice-articulation modification in people with neurological disorders have also tempered unmodified wholesale adoption of sports science principles. People have questioned whether relearning after brain injury happens in the same way as in a healthy brain, whether cognitive-motor skills required for speech are comparable to those needed for the kinds of actions studied in the general motor learning literature. Speech is not just infinitely more complex than most of these simpler tasks; the patterns of movement control can vary greatly too (Kent, 2004; Maas, 2017; Ziegler & Ackermann, 2013).

Much of sports learning is directed at faster, higher and stronger. But, do faster, stronger articulatory muscles necessarily lead to improved speech intelligibility? The rationale for oral gymnastic exercises is that in dysarthria, muscles are weak and slow, therefore drills to effect stronger, faster, further must be a benefit. There is some evidence that increases in selected movements of the articulators are possible from simple oral gymnastics (Clark, 2008; Kent, 2015; Mackenzie et al., 2014). However, it is far from settled whether or how these gains translate into improved speech, greater intelligibility and more successful communication.

At least two observations appear to explain why not. First, successful speech movements require only a small fraction of the maximum force that these muscles are capable of (Whitwell et al., 2019), so, for weakness to be a main factor in reduced speech skills demands severe impairment.

Second, speech is not controlled on an articulator-by-articulator basis but on simultaneous integration of overlapping, ennested and entrained movements and adjustments across the whole vocal tract to signal sound contrasts. Training movements, not part of speech and/or variables isolated from the whole, risks practising movements in ways that do not happen in speech and in a manner of control (isolated not integrated) that does not reflect reality. Targeting sounds in isolation ignores that in real life, sounds only ever occur in contrast with each other. At the least, neglecting these truisms adds unnecessary stages in therapy; at the worst, such exercises prove entirely counterproductive.

These arguments underpin assertions that to improve speech, one practises only verbal tasks. It is by smithying that one becomes a blacksmith, so the French proverb goes. One needs strong muscles, certainly, but these come from practising what smithies do. Non-verbal drills such as silently opening and closing the lips, blowing a ping-pong ball across the table, shooting the tongue in and out or side to side do not involve patterns of movement and control that occur in speech.

A perspective that favours overall integration across the whole vocal tract shifts the search for what is important in intervention to finding tasks/instructions/strategies that preserve integration across the vocal tract, achieve simultaneous reorganisation of related variables and exploit the wholistic control of voice–speech sound production and perception. This is why findings (given previously) indicating the efficacy of interventions such as attention to effort, rate control and prosody manipulation that preserve movements across the whole vocal tract are so exciting. Furthermore, relying on a single input (slower; louder; stronger, etc.) applied to the entire speech act means instructions are cognitively and mechanically straightforward. They require attention to a single dimension. They bypass potentially complex therapist centred instructions on how to move the articulators. They leave the speaker to find their own solution to arrive at the target. This brings us to the critical topic of feedback.

Instructions and feedback

Crucial variables around how frequently, what on and how one delivers feedback influence motor learning (Bakker, Beijer, & Rietveld, 2019; Schmidt et al., 2018; Shumway-Cook & Woollacott, 2016). Space precludes elucidation of all the issues here (speech versus non-speech, neurologically healthy versus impaired, etc.). Two central points concern the scheduling of feedback and what feedback draws attention to.

Feedback scheduling

Feedback after every attempt (or every second, third, etc.) facilitates more rapid (re)acquisition of a specific task but leaves learning vulnerable to relapse after withdrawal of feedback and poor generalisation to related behaviours. Less frequent and more irregular feedback may slow (re)acquisition but favours maintenance and generalisation. For people with dysarthria, the recommendation then appears to be to commence with frequent regular, extrinsic (from clinician or device) feedback but gradually phase this out to less frequent, irregular and eventually to the speaker's own internal, intrinsic monitoring.

Feedback on what?

There are several issues. One central distinction concerns whether feedback informs speaker internal processes, the movements they are using to reach the target, versus external, result-oriented outcomes and how successful their effort sounds. Specific, speaker internal, feedback might be 'raise the back of your tongue'; 'make your tongue flatter' and 'make sure the air comes through your nose'. External, result-oriented feedback examples might be: 'Don't forget the sound at the end of the word'; 'it still sounded too much like 'mine' not 'wine' and 'do it louder so the neighbours hear'.

Both forms play a role. Internal, process feedback works if manipulation of one parameter will make the crucial difference to performance. It succeeds only if the speaker can actually isolate and control the variable within the general stream of movement. If movements are not accessible to manipulation and voluntary control (e.g. velum raising and voice onset time), the speaker cannot hear/feel the target difference and/or feedback is too complicated ('raise your tongue tip behind your top teeth but make sure it still lets some air through with your tongue grooved and have your vocal cords vibrating'), then such feedback becomes self-defeating. The advantage of an external focus is that it permits individuals to find their own solution by manipulating proprioceptive, kinaesthetic variables they themselves can control, within the context of reorganisation of the whole vocal tract. Both forms of feedback presume the speaker knows what they are aiming for, reiterating the importance of preparatory watch and listen work where the speaker hears and sees what the target is, followed by unison practice with the clinician or device.

Conclusion

Dysarthria represents a disorder of speech that arises against the backdrop of highly diverse medical, cognitive, age, social and rehabilitation circumstances. These dictate a necessarily varied approach to management. The evidence base for dysarthria assessment and management is not as well developed as other fields, and despite some systematic reviews in selected areas of the topic in recent years, much decision-making still relies on clinical experience and expert opinion. Nonetheless, there are solid theoretical principles and clinical guidelines on which dysarthria management should be based. The cases in the upcoming chapters delve into application of these in a variety of common clinical scenarios.

References

Bakker, M., Beijer, L., & Rietveld, T. (2019). Considerations on effective feedback in computerized speech training for dysarthric speakers. *Telemedicine and e-Health, 25*(5), 351–358. doi:10.1089/tmj.2018.0050

Ballard, K. J., Wambaugh, J. L., Duffy, J. R., Layfield, C., Maas, E., Mauszycki, S., & McNeil, M. R. (2015). Treatment for acquired apraxia of speech: A systematic review of intervention research between 2004 and 2012. *American Journal of Speech-Language Pathology, 24*(2), 316–337. doi:10.1044/2015_AJSLP-14-0118

Chiu, Y.-F., & Neel, A. (2020). Predicting intelligibility deficits in Parkinson's disease with perceptual speech ratings. *Journal of Speech, Language, & Hearing Research, 63*(2), 433–443. doi:10.1044/2019_JSLHR-19-00134

Clark, H. M. (2008). The role of strength training in speech sound disorders. *Seminars in Speech and Language, 29*(4), 276–283. doi:10.1055/s-0028-1103391

Coleman, A., Weir, K., Ware, R. S., & Boyd, R. (2015). Predicting functional communication ability in children with cerebral palsy at school entry. *Developmental Medicine and Child Neurology, 57*(3), 279–285. doi:10.1111/dmcn.12631

Dobinson, C., & Miller, N. (2019). Does my intervention make a difference to my client's impairment? In C. Dobinson & Y. Wren (Eds.), *Creating practice-based evidence* (pp. 153–181). London: J&R Press.

Duffy, J. (2019). *Motor speech disorders* (4th ed.). St. Louis: Mosby Elsevier.

Finch, E., Rumbach, A. F., & Park, S. (2020). Speech pathology management of non-progressive dysarthria: A systematic review of the literature. *Disability and Rehabilitation, 42*(3), 296–306. doi:10.1080/09638288.2018.1497714

Gillivan-Murphy, P., Miller, N., & Carding, P. (2019). Voice treatment in Parkinson's disease: Patient perspectives. *Research and Reviews in Parkinsonism, 9,* 29–42.

Gustafsson, J. K., Södersten, M., Ternström, S., & Schalling, E. (2019). Voice use in daily life studied with a portable voice accumulator in individuals with Parkinson's disease and matched healthy controls. *Journal of Speech, Language and Hearing Research, 62*(12), 4324–4334. doi:10.1044/2019_JSLHR-19-00037

Hartelius, L., & Miller, N. (2010). The ICF framework and its relevance to the assessment of people with motor speech disorders. In L. Lowit & R. Kent (Eds.), *Assessment of motor speech disorders.* San Diego, CA: Plural.

Hixon, T., Weismer, G., & Holt, J. (2008). *Preclinical speech science.* San Diego, CA: Plural.

Kent, R. (2004). The uniqueness of speech among motor systems. *Clinical Linguistics & Phonetics, 18*(6–8), 495–505. Retrieved from <Go to ISI>://000225105200011

Kent, R. (2015). Nonspeech oral movements and oral motor disorders: A narrative review. *American Journal of Speech-Language Pathology, 24*(4), 763–789. doi:10.1044/2015_AJSLP-14-0179

Kuschmann, A., Miller, N., Lowit, A., & Pennington, L. (2017). Intonation patterns in older children with cerebral palsy before and after speech intervention. *International Journal of Speech-Language Pathology, 19*(4), 370–380. doi:10.1080/17549507.2016.1216601

Lousada, M., Jesus, L. M. T., Hall, A., & Joffe, V. (2014). Intelligibility as a clinical outcome measure following intervention with children with phonologically based speech-sound disorders. *International Journal of Language & Communication Disorders, 49*(5), 584–601. doi:10.1111/1460-6984.12095

Lowit, A., & Kent, R. (Eds.). (2011). *Assessment of motor speech disorders.* San Diego, CA: Singular.

Maas, E. (2017). Speech and nonspeech: What are we talking about? *International Journal of Speech-Language Pathology, 19*(4), 345–359. doi:10.1080/17549507.2016.1221995

Mackenzie, C., Muir, M., Allen, C., & Jensen, A. (2014). Non-speech oro-motor exercises in post-stroke dysarthria intervention: A randomized feasibility trial. *International Journal of Language & Communication Disorders, 49*(5), 602–617. doi:10.1111/1460-6984.12096

McAuliffe, M. J., Baylor, C. R., & Yorkston, K. M. (2017). Variables associated with communicative participation in Parkinson's disease and its relationship to measures of health-related quality-of-life. *International Journal of Speech-Language Pathology, 19*(4), 407–417. doi:10.1080/17549507.2016.1193900

McAuliffe, M. J., Fletcher, A. R., Kerr, S. E., O'Beirne, G. A., & Anderson, T. (2017). Effect of dysarthria type, speaking condition, and listener age on speech intelligibility. *American Journal of Speech-Language Pathology, 26*(1), 113–123. doi:10.1044/2016_AJSLP-15-0182

Miller, N. (2013). Measuring up to speech intelligibility. *International Journal of Language & Communication Disorders, 46*(6), 613–624.

Miller, N. (2017). Communication changes in Parkinson's disease. *Practical Neurology, 17*(4), 266–274. doi:10.1136/practneurol-2017-001635

Miller, N., Allcock, L., Jones, D., Noble, E., Hildreth, A. J., & Burn, D. J. (2007). Prevalence and pattern of perceived intelligibility changes in Parkinson's disease. *Journal of Neurology, Neurosurgery & Psychiatry, 78*(11), 1188–1190. doi:10.1136/jnnp.2006.110171

Miller, N., & Bloch, S. (2017). A survey of speech-language therapy provision for people with post-stroke dysarthria in the UK. *International Journal of Language & Communication Disorders*, *52*(6), 800–815. doi:10.1111/1460-6984.12316

Miller, N., & Lowit, A. (Eds.). (2014). *Motor speech disorders: A cross language perspective.* Clevedon: Multilingual Matters.

Miller, N., Nath, U., Noble, E., & Burn, D. (2017). Utility and accuracy of perceptual voice and speech distinctions in the diagnosis of Parkinson's disease, Progressive Supranuclear Palsy and Multiple System Atrophy with prominent Parkinson's. *Neurodegenerative Disease Management*, *7*(3). https://doi.org/10.2217/nmt-2017-0005

Miller, N., Noble, E., Jones, D., Allcock, L., & Burn, D. J. (2008). How do I sound to me? Perceived changes in communication in Parkinson's disease. *Clinical Rehabilitation*, *22*(1), 14–22. doi:10.1177/0269215507079096

Miller, N., Noble, E., Jones, D., Deane, K. H. O., & Gibb, C. (2011). Survey of speech and language therapy provision for people with Parkinson's disease in the United Kingdom: Patients' and carers' perspectives. *International Journal of Language & Communication Disorders*, *46*(2), 179–188. doi:10.3109/13682822.2010.484850

Miller, N., & Wambaugh, J. (2021). Apraxia of speech: Nature, assessment, treatment. In I. Papathanasiou & P. Coppens (Eds.), *Aphasia and related neurogenic communication disorders* (3rd ed., pp. 603–640). Boston, MA: Jones & Bartlett.

Mitchell, C., Bowen, A., Tyson, S., Butterfint, Z., & Conroy, P. (2017). Interventions for dysarthria due to stroke and other adult-acquired, non-progressive brain injury. *Cochrane Database of Systematic Reviews*, *1*. doi:10.1002/14651858.CD002088.pub3

Munoz-Vigueras, N., Prados-Roman, E., Valenza, M. C., Granados-Santiago, M., Cabrera-Martos, I., Rodriguez-Torres, J., & Torres-Sanchez, I. (2020). Speech and language therapy treatment on hypokinetic dysarthria in Parkinson disease: Systematic review and meta-analysis. *Clinical Rehabilitation*, 269215520976267–269215520976267. doi:10.1177/0269215520976267

Noffs, G., Perera, T., Kolbe, S. C., Shanahan, C. J., Boonstra, F. M. C., Evans, A., . . . Vogel, A. P. (2018). What speech can tell us: A systematic review of dysarthria characteristics in multiple sclerosis. *Autoimmunity Reviews*, *17*(12), 1202–1209. doi:10.1016/j.autrev.2018.06.010

Palmer, A. D., Carder, P. C., White, D. L., Saunders, G., Woo, H., Graville, D. J., & Newsom, J. T. (2019). The impact of communication impairments on the social relationships of older adults: Pathways to psychological well-being. *Journal of Speech Language & Hearing Research*, *62*(1), 1–21. doi:10.1044/2018_jslhr-s-17-0495

Park, S., Theodoros, D., Finch, E., & Cardell, E. (2016). Be clear: A new intensive speech treatment for adults with nonprogressive dysarthria. *American Journal of Speech-Language Pathology*, *25*(1), 97–110. doi:10.1044/2015_AJSLP-14-0113

Patel, R., Connaghan, K. P., & Campellone, P. J. (2013). The effect of rate reduction on signaling prosodic contrasts in dysarthria. *Folia Phoniatrica*, *65*(3), 109–116. doi:10.1159/000354422

Pennington, L., Miller, N., Robson, S., & Steen, N. (2010). Intensive speech and language therapy for older children with cerebral palsy: A systems approach. *Developmental Medicine & Child Neurology*, *52*(4), 337–344. http://dx.doi.org/10.1111/j.1469-8749.2009.03366.x

Read, J. L., Whittaker, R. G., Miller, N., Clark, S., Taylor, R., McFarland, R., & Turnbull, D. (2012). Prevalence and severity of voice and swallowing difficulties in mitochondrial disease. *International Journal of Language & Communication Disorders*, *47*(1), 106–111. doi:10.1111/j.1460-6984.2011.00072.x

Sackley, C., Rick, C., Au, P., Brady, M., Beaton, G., Burton, C., . . . Clarke, C. (2020). A multicentre, randomised controlled trial to compare the clinical and cost-effectiveness of Lee Silverman Voice Treatment versus standard NHS speech and language therapy versus control in Parkinson's disease: A study protocol for a randomised controlled trial. *Trials, 21*(1). doi:10.1186/s13063-020-04354-7

Schalling, E., Johansson, K., & Hartelius, L. (2017). Speech and communication changes reported by people with Parkinson's disease. *Folia Phoniatrica, 69*(3), 131–141. www.karger.com/DOI/10.1159/000479927

Schmidt, R. A., Lee, T. D., Winstein, C., Wulf, G., & Zelaznik, H. N. (2018). *Motor control and learning: A behavioral emphasis.* New York: Human Kinetics.

Sescleifer, A. M., Francoisse, C. A., & Lin, A. Y. (2018). Systematic review: Online crowd-sourcing to assess perceptual speech outcomes. *Journal of Surgical Research, 232,* 351–364. doi:10.1016/j.jss.2018.06.032

Shumway-Cook, A., & Woollacott, M. H. (2016). *Motor control: Translating research into clinical practice* (5th ed.). Philadelphia: Lippincott Williams & Wilkins.

Tan, S., van Gorp, M., Voorman, J., Geytenbeek, J., Reinders-Messelink, H., Ketelaar, M., . . . Roebroeck, M. (2020). Development curves of communication and social interaction in individuals with cerebral palsy. *Developmental Medicine and Child Neurology, 62*(1), 132–139. doi:10.1111/dmcn.14351

Vieira, H., Costa, N., Sousa, T., Reis, S., & Coelho, L. (2020). Voice-based classification of amyotrophic lateral sclerosis: Where are we and where are we going? Systematic review. *Neurodegenerative Diseases, 19*(5–6), 163–170. doi:10.1159/000506259

Walshe, M., & Miller, N. (2011). Living with acquired dysarthria: The speaker's perspective. *Disability and Rehabilitation, 33*(3), 195–203. doi:10.3109/09638288.2010.511685

Walshe, M., Miller, N., Leahy, M., & Murray, A. (2008). Intelligibility of dysarthric speech: Perceptions of speakers and listeners. *International Journal of Language & Communication Disorders, 43*(6), 633–648. doi:10.1080/13682820801887117

Wannberg, P., Schalling, E., & Hartelius, L. (2016). Perceptual assessment of dysarthria: Comparison of a general and a detailed assessment protocol. *Logopedics Phoniatrics Vocology, 41*(4), 159–167. doi:10.3109/14015439.2015.1069889

Whillans, C., Lawrie, M., Cardell, E. A., Kelly, C., & Wenke, R. (2020). A systematic review of group intervention for acquired dysarthria in adults. *Disability & Rehabilitation.* doi:10.1080/09638288.2020.1859629

Whitwell, J. L., Stevens, C. A., Duffy, J. R., Clark, H. M., Machulda, M. M., Strand, E. A., . . . Josephs, K. A. (2019). An evaluation of the progressive supranuclear palsy speech/language variant. *Movement Disorders Clinical Practice, 6*(6), 452–461. doi:10.1002/mdc3.12796

Wight, S., & Miller, N. (2015). Lee Silverman Voice Treatment for people with Parkinson's: Audit of outcomes in a routine clinic. *International Journal of Language & Communication Disorders, 50*(2), 215–225. doi:10.1111/1460-6984.12132

Wray, F., & Clarke, D. (2017). Longer-term needs of stroke survivors with communication difficulties living in the community: A systematic review and thematic synthesis of qualitative studies. *BMJ Open, 7*(10). doi:10.1136/bmjopen-2017-017944

Wray, F., Clarke, D., & Forster, A. (2019). How do stroke survivors with communication difficulties manage life after stroke in the first year? A qualitative study. *International Journal of Language & Communication Disorders, 54*(5), 814–827. doi:10.1111/1460-6984.12487

Yorkston, K., Baylor, C., & Britton, D. (2017). Incorporating the principles of self-management into treatment of dysarthria associated with Parkinson's disease. *Seminars in Speech and Language, 38*(3), 210–219. doi:10.1055/s-0037-1602840

Yuan, F., Guo, X., Wei, X., Xie, F., Zheng, J., Huang, Y., . . . Wang, Q. (2020). Lee Silverman Voice Treatment for dysarthria in patients with Parkinson's disease: A systematic review and meta-analysis. *European Journal of Neurology, 27*(10), 1957–1970. doi:10.1111/ene.14399

Ziegler, W., & Ackermann, H. (2013). Neuromotor speech impairment: It's all in the talking. *Folia Phoniatric, 65*(2), 55–67. doi:10.1159/000353855

Chapter 2

A trip up the garden path

Functional speech disorders

Nick Miller

Introduction

Day-to-day cases in the speech clinic generally follow fairly predictable lines, even if some are clearly more complex and demand considerable expertise to disentangle all the factors at play in assessment and management. There are, though, instances where what appears straightforward at first sight turns out to be anything but. Such cases are not so rare as we might think. This chapter looks at such a case.

General background

Paula (a pseudonym) was 45 years old. Her family doctor referred her to speech-language therapy/pathology (SLT/SLP) because she was troubled by her speech since a short hospitalisation four weeks previously.

She answered general case history questions directly and appropriately. She had a teenage girl and boy and husband (waiting outside in the car, preferring not to come in). She grew up locally and worked full-time as a secretary in a large road transport firm since leaving school aged 18. Leisure time activities centred largely around reading, TV and meeting friends. She was right-handed, reported no hearing problems, but wore glasses for reading and computer. She smoked 15–20 cigarettes a day and drank around 15 units of alcohol per week. Paula explained the cane she was using helped with some right leg weakness, which, she said, came from her recent stroke. Apart from this, she volunteered no past or present surgical, medical, psychiatric or psychological issues that she felt relevant. Probed further, she mentioned recurrent migraines.

These started in her early 20s, occurring a few times a year, but did not restrict her life. Over the past 10–15 years, they had become progressively more frequent (now around one per month) and severe – anything from 'a blinding headache', off work for the day, to needing to lie in darkness for several days. On three occasions she was hospitalised with hemiplegic migraines (www. migrainetrust.org/about-migraine/types-of-migraine/hemiplegic-migraine/

DOI: 10.4324/9781003172536-2

accessed 7 June 2021). These lasted up to 24–36 hours, with flashing lights, hemi-weakness and slurred speech. They occasioned referral to a neurologist who prescribed topiramate 2 × 25 mg/day.

Paula reported that the recent stroke started as what felt like another hemiplegic migraine, with accompanying speech changes. She spent three days in hospital. This time, unlike previously, when the migraine resolved, her hemiplegia and speech did not recover. She felt her arm and leg weakness had improved over the last month, but not her speech. This, and how people reacted to it, was upsetting. It was affecting her daily living and returning to work. She had lost confidence speaking and feared clients would not understand her. Hence, her request for referral to SLT/SLP. She had never attended SLT/SLP before. Although speech changes accompanied the hemiplegic migraines, they always cleared when it did.

Her speech: first impressions

Impressionistically, output sounded disordered. Voice quality was mildly asthenic (1 on Asthenia scale of GRBAS (DeBodt, Wuyts, VandeHeyning, & Croux, 1997) though Paula described herself as never a loud speaker. Intonation and loudness variation seemed restricted, though by no means completely monotone or monoloud. Was this maybe early onset Parkinson's disease? (Miller, 2017). Several unexpected exaggerated rises and falls in intonation, and stress placed on the wrong syllable in a word or sentence seemed to discount this. She said 'roundAbout' for the road-junction and 'we came IN THE car today', not the expected 'ROUNdabout' and 'we CAme in the CAR today'. Output contained hesitations, apparent difficulties initiating phonation or blocking on a sound and repeated sounds or syllables. Diagnostically, thoughts of acquired stuttering arose.

Resonance sounded normal, except for intermittent distinctly hypernasal utterances leading to what her husband later described as 'her French voice'. Could this be foreign accent syndrome? (McWhirter et al., 2019; Ryalls & Miller, 2014).

Sounds were certainly distorted, sufficient sometimes to affect intelligibility and for her to need to repeat. On general listening, no manner or place of articulation sounded to be selectively affected. Indeed, sound production appeared somewhat inconsistent – the same sound was not always distorted or was distorted in a different way. The dysfluencies, inconsistent realisation of sounds and misplacement of word and sentence stress prompted thoughts that this might be AOS (apraxia of speech) or dysarthria plus AOS (Miller & Wambaugh, 2021).

There were no red flags for dysphagia, no changes to ease of eating/drinking or time taken for meals and no changes to foodstuffs or drinks she could manage. There was no observed or reported sialorrhea.

General motor status, apart from her balance/walking, appeared unremarkable. Facial expression was effortless, appropriate and without obvious asymmetry. Occasionally, when struggling on an apparently blocked sound, her face contorted. Paula reported no sensory perceptual or neuropsychological sequelae from the hospital episode. She described herself as 'happy enough', apart from frustration at the speech changes and how people reacted negatively to these.

During case history taking, apart from sometimes impaired intelligibility, she conveyed her thoughts clearly. However, there were circumlocutions and possible semantic and phonological paraphasias. Paula was aware of these. She called 'stairs' the 'going-up steps', described where the 'motorbike' (not car) was parked and named her ['dozetə] (daughter) and ['hubent] (husband). So, there might be mild aphasia, an idea strengthened by some unusual grammatical constructions – for example, 'we are coming out the house at a 9.30' (expected utterance: we came out/left the house at 9.30), 'my husband downstair he is yes waiting' (expected reply: (yes) my husband is waiting downstairs). Such instances had caused raised voices between Paula and her husband when he could not work out what she was trying to express.

Formal assessment

Assessment followed a week later to fix baseline measures and establish a differential diagnosis. At this stage, the working hypothesis was AOS, based on the seeming lack of significant weakness but nevertheless disordered articulation characterised by inconsistency, dysprosody and dysfluency (Miller & Wambaugh, 2021). However, given the altered voice quality and stretches of hypernasal resonance, dysarthria was not excluded. The possible paraphasias and atypical grammar suggested screening for aphasia. The referral letter mentioned no medical history aside from recent hospitalisation, so full medical reports were obtained. As Paula had alluded to issues with listeners, including her husband, this was pursued.

Motor speech and intelligibility examination followed the scheme outlined in Table 1.1 (see Chapter 1). Since AOS was suspected, various supplementary tasks (Table 2.1) looked at the type and quantity of sound derailments across variables that help distinguish dysarthria from AOS.

The aphasia screen consisted of a naming test (Kaplan, Goodglass, & Weintraub, 2001) and speeded naming by category, and starting with letters F, A and S (Whiteside et al., 2016). The grammaticality judgement task and lexicality task of SCOLP (Baddeley, Emslie, & Nimmo-Smith, 1992) looked at speed and accuracy of language processing and estimated premorbid verbal intelligence. Describing the Boston Cookie Theft picture (Goodglass & Kaplan, 2001), explaining how to make a cup of tea and reading the Grandfather Passage (Reilly & Fisher, 2012) provided data for analysis of motor speech features in connected speech and possible aphasia signs.

Table 2.1 Rules of thumb to aid distinction of dysarthria from AOS

	Dysarthria	AOS
Respiration, phonation	Affected by hypertonic or hypotonic cords, reduced subglottal pressure and/or discoordination of respiration–phonation	Voice changes unlikely to be a major factor; maybe affected by voice initiation difficulty and hypertonic voice during struggle episodes
Resonance	If velum impaired, possible hypernasality	Hypernasality unlikely a problem; maybe occasional 'substitution' of nasal–oral cognates
Diadochokinesis (DDK)	Over repetitions, rate slows, target contacts weaken and sound contrasts fade – for example, *tea-sea* sounds like *sea-sea* or *he-he*	Difficulties attaining and staying on target and keeping consistent target order, rhythm and stress. Possible effortful, trial-and-error self-corrections
Non-verbal DDK	Derailment quality and quantity correlate across ±verbal tasks	Errors in the absence of neuromuscular changes or speech error rate out of proportion to severity of any neuromuscular changes
Increasing syllables	For example, do/dew-duty-dutiful. Longer more likely in error in dysarthria and AOS. Dysarthric distortions more likely from range/force difficulties	Distortions more likely reflect discoordination between articulators, inconsistent realisation of specific sounds across words and metathetic errors, for example, citizen sounds like tisizen
Increasing complexity	For example, A-pay-play-plate-plates. Longer more likely in error in dysarthria and AOS. Dysarthria more likely range/force, sustainability difficulties	AOS movement coordination and consistency issues; metathetic errors possible. Cross-syllable consonant clusters particularly prone, for example, dogbone sounds like dogubbone; witchcraft like *twichcaf*
±Overlearned sequences	Little effect on error rate, for example, 12345 versus 54321	More overlearned (days, counting and prayers) less errorful than same words in non-overlearned context/order (art, heaven and father)
Frequency effect	Little effect on errors, for example, *play* versus *ploy*	Low frequency words more likely in error
Sense–nonsense words	Little effect on errors, for example, *play* versus *ploo*	Nonsense words more error-prone
Prosody	Generally, rate slowed, fundamental frequency range reduced, intensity envelope reduced and in ataxic dysarthria, possible scanning rhythm	Rate generally slowed. Non-canonical stress patterns more likely trigger errors; presence of excessive or wrong intonation/stress patterns and dysfluencies (blocks, hesitations and repetitions)

To gauge how far Paula's feeling of self as a communicator had altered since before the speech changes, she completed a semantic differential questionnaire (Miller, Noble, Jones, Allcock, & Burn, 2008) and dysarthria impact profile (Atkinson-Clement et al., 2019; Walshe, Peach, & Miller, 2009).

Results

The impact questionnaires indicated social intercourse had shrunk considerably. Paula still felt herself intelligent, with worthy things to contribute, but her confidence in communicating had sunk compared to previously and anxiety over reactions of others to her speech was a big concern.

On the surface, a diagnosis of AOS and mild aphasia was tempting. Segmental and prosodic derailments arose in the presence of no obvious difficulty with range, force and rate of movements. Misarticulations appeared linked to difficulties coordinating across multiple subsystems (e.g. tongue-tip with tongue-back, phonation-articulation and nasal–oral articulation). 'Paraphasias' and atypical syntax heard in case history taking arose.

There was, though, an unease about the picture. Paula's realisations were certainly inconsistent, and many distortions could be interpreted as instances of miscoordination across subsystems – both characteristics of AOS. However, closer scrutiny revealed details not compatible with AOS (Table 2.1). Quantitative scores were not the key issue. Rather, the qualitative discrepancies and incongruities between and within tests alerted to a different diagnosis.

Whilst misarticulations of the type below occurred in the first meeting and led to suspicions of AOS, formal assessment showed that likelihood of derailment did not vary in relation to either length or complexity, word frequency, nor rate of articulation. She evidenced greater difficulty with selected longer and more complex words and phrases, but tellingly read many of them relatively effortlessly whilst stumbling on articulatorily simple, high-frequency sounds and syllables. 'Eight mechanics fixed Jake's tractor' and 'That magician's tricks seemed like witchcraft', deemed complex, were heard as ['eimə'xanı'fisʃeikˀ'tratə] and [ʃmə'ʒıʃəntrı'simlaı 'wıʃɹæf]. However 'I put a packet by the cupboard' and 'Buy Bobby a poppy today Katy', considered simple, became [æ:.'æ:m:'bwu:dz.'wu:dz'pætʃt'mba:hə.'ba'kxʊbz], and [keı'baı.baı.m:hə'baı.'boʔ'bob.bı'pa: pı'deı/. Thus, rather than a positive frequency/complexity effect, whether derailments occurred across these gradients approached chance.

There were further instances where Paula seemed to experience difficulties with some (af)fricatives, along with vowel distortions – for example, from the Cookie Theft description: [zi'sizə'boıonzi'ʃeə] (this is a/the boy on the chair). Like her intermittent hypernasality, this conveyed the impression of a pseudo-French accent – pseudo since she had no association with French accents previously, 'Frenchness' emerged only intermittently, not pervasively, and without displaying other characteristics of how French speakers might pronounce English.

Incongruencies also emerged on DDK tasks. Paula struggled to produce ten repetitions of 'tea-D' yet later managed 'pea-tea-key' accurately and effortlessly, and in her spontaneous speech and reading distinguishing /ti-di/, and other voiced-voiceless pairs seldom appeared an issue. Furthermore, when producing 'tea-D' as fast as possible, her apparent difficulty seemed to be range and rate of movement despite full-range movements on other challenge tasks.

A comparable picture materialised when listening for resonance changes. People with AOS may produce what sounds like nasal/oral substitutions – /mʊk/ for /bʊk/, 'nine' as /daɪd/, /daɪnd/ or /ndaɪd/. No such instances happened. Instead, similar to how range (previous paragraph) difficulty seemed to be then not be a problem, hypernasal speech occurred for a phrase (or few), but then was fine again. Such performance is inconsistent with AOS and most dysarthria manifestations. Dystonia may sometimes produce such transitory disruptions, but no other signs or symptoms pointed to dystonia.

Similar inconsistencies characterised the performance on the aphasia screens. There were misnamings and some delayed responses on the naming test. These did not clearly correlate with any indices of visual or articulatory frequency and complexity. Speeded naming by category or letter was typified by apparent articulatory and mind blocks ('my mind's gone blank'). Her 90th percentile attainment on the SCOLP Spot-the-Word test suggested good pre-morbid and current verbal ability. It contrasted starkly with her 25th percentile score on sentence processing. This came not from pervasive slowness and/or error responses but from puzzling long over the answer (yes/no) on just a few items (e.g. Jeeps are vehicles; melons are people) despite readily judging similar sentences successfully (e.g. chests of drawers wear clothes).

The nature of the articulatory derailments, the random, not rule-governed, likelihood of misarticulations and misnamings and irregular syntactic stumblings all seemed to refute that AOS and aphasia were key problems. The same went for dysarthria. So, was this some atypical presentation of AOS, aphasia and/or dysarthria? If so, why and in what way?

There are many mimics of stroke or strokes masquerading under other guises (Fernandes, Whiteley, Hart, & Al-Shahi Salman, 2013; Nadarajan, Perry, Johnson, & Werring, 2014). Are the hemiplegic migraines maybe some complicating factor that makes an otherwise typical stroke presentation atypical? Is the apparent spontaneous recovery of the hemiplegia but not of speech a clue? If so, a clue for what? Maybe the handedness assessment was insufficiently thorough and this is an example of crossed aphasia/AOS (Assal, Laganaro, Remund, & Paquier, 2012; Marien, Paghera, De Deyn, & Vignolo, 2004)? Was this perhaps the early presentation of some progressive neurological condition so far manifesting only in speech (Miller, Nath, Noble, & Burn, 2017; Montembeault, Brambati, Gorno-Tempini, & Migliaccio, 2018; Takakura et al., 2019)? If so, which one, and what other clues should we look for? Alternatively, was Paula presenting with a functional speech disorder?

Functional speech disorders

Though functional *speech* changes have received less attention, functional disorders frequently appear in the speech clinic (Baker et al., 2021; Chung, Wettroth, Hallett, & Maurer, 2018; Espay et al., 2018; Mendez, 2018). Manifestations include (s)elective mutism, certain forms of voice disorder and altered resonance (e.g. functional falsetto, infantilisms and pharynge-alisation), acquired functional dysfluency, speech affectations (e.g. sniffs and drawling) and functional foreign accent syndrome (McWhirter et al., 2019; Romö, Miller, & Cardoso, 2021; Ryalls & Miller, 2014).

Functional neurological symptom disorders straddle the border between neurology and psychiatry. They represent cases with neurological-like symptoms (e.g. weakness, tremor, dyskinesia, seizures, dysphagia, word finding and syntax difficulties) where thorough investigation reveals no disease, trauma, or structural abnormalities that account for them. Observation shows patterns of behaviour inconsistent with structural, neurological changes. Nonetheless, the changes and consequences experienced by individuals are as real, distressing and disabling as neurological aetiologies, and not to be dismissed lightly.

Functional disorders are not synonymous with feigning, malingering or facti-tious disorder. Simply hearing 'bizarre' speech/voice is not indicative of functional aetiology – neurological disorders can cause highly unusual behaviours. Speech–voice alterations accompany some psychiatric conditions, but diagnosing psychiatric dysfunction is not prerequisite to establishing functional disorders (Espay et al., 2018). Furthermore, neurological and functional disorders may coexist. The relationship need not be cause and effect. The clinician's task is to untangle which behaviours relate to the neurological changes and which to the functional disorders.

Differentiation rests on an intimate knowledge of the causes, course, range of presenting symptoms and their variation, associated with candidate syn-dromes. Diagnosis, however, does not rest solely on ruling out all other pos-sibilities, and functional neurological disorders should be recognisable by positive, rule-in features.

Recognising functional speech disorders

Various rule-in possibilities have been suggested (Baker et al., 2021; Chung et al., 2018; McWhirter et al., 2019; Mendez, 2018; Romö et al., 2021). Table 2.2 summarises some of them. No feature alone confirms/refutes a functional diagnosis. Accumulation of pointers on the one side of the chart or the other and interpretation of the communication picture in the context of wider neu-rological, physical, psychological and social assessment guides differentiation. Key features concern inconsistency in how and when behaviours/symptoms occur and lack of congruence between observed behaviours and known pat-terns and consequences of neurological conditions (Romö et al., 2021).

Table 2.2 Selected rules of thumb for differentiating functional from neurological voice–
        speech disturbance

Points more to functional	Points more to neurological
Presenting signs and symptoms do not fit known neurological syndromes	Presenting signs and symptoms fall into familiar neurological clusters
Speech characteristics incongruent with the presenting physical/structural picture	Close tie between the severity and loci of physical/structural changes and speech profile
Speech presentation varies according to the person, place, topic, especially where any of these is linked to emotionally loaded factors	Speech varies according to fatigue, recognised drug effects and well-known linguistic parameters (e.g. automaticity, word class and frequency effects and syllable structure)
Apparently random, unexplainable variation in severity or symptoms; symptoms described as linked vary independently of one another. Possible reversibility of symptoms	Variation follows lawful patterns linked to known physiological, language and speech production/perception effects
Sudden onset associated with significant life or other precipitating event	Sudden onset associated with demonstrable neurological event
Gradual onset associated with build-up of negative life events or other stressful precipitating situation(s)	Gradual onset independent of other life events; follows onset pattern of known neurological illnesses
Predisposing/perpetuating/risk factors and comorbidities more likely overlap with affective, psychosocial and personality domains	Predisposing/perpetuating/risk variables and comorbidities more likely reflect factors closely associated with stroke and neurological disorders

Did Paula have a functional disorder?

The principal deciders in concluding a functional disorder for Paula centred on: (a) the incongruity/disconnection between her speech symptoms and intact underlying speech motor status, (b) inconsistency (across time and within conversations across words) in which specific speech and language changes arose and (c) lack of explanatory accounts for speech–voice changes within the framework of known neurological motor speech disorders.

Paula's husband revealed more relevant material. This was not the first time Paula had experienced speech changes independent of her migraines. The family had witnessed unintelligible articulation and/or inappropriate misnaming and sentence structure intermittently for several years. They had heard episodes (a few words, sometimes many sentences) of hypernasal speech that family and friends branded her 'French voice'. Her husband reacted with embarrassment in case she spoke like this outside and, as he had expressed to her several times, by telling her to stop, she did not need to talk like that or attract attention to herself. This caused tension between them, since Paula felt no power to control or modify her speech.

The hospital reports supported functional aetiology. Brain imaging had found no evidence of stroke, neoplasm or progressive conditions. Paula was nevertheless convinced she had a stroke. Regardless of contrary evidence, she felt this was just more of people fobbing her off, not believing her, even deceiving her. She had consulted a solicitor over suing the hospital for negligence, in not recognising her 'stroke'. The solicitor declined the case. This only fuelled her feeling of people not taking her seriously.

Why did she have a functional disorder?

Functional disorders may have a clear onset and/or trigger. More commonly, the onset is insidious; contributing factors are multiple, complex and unclear. Speakers themselves may have no idea of specific factors. This was true for Paula. However, some tentative insights Paula ventured during intervention led her to contemplate possible influences.

She left school aged 18, but believed she could have succeeded in higher education, like her husband. Work was agreeable, but she resented being bottom of the pile, the scapegoat when things went awry. She was demoralised being regularly overlooked for promotion, despite her initial confidence that she could go far in the firm. Paula drew parallels between this and how she often felt treated at home – sacrificing her ambitions for the family, playing second string to her successful husband, not being taken seriously. She worried about the children's schooling and whether they might get into drugs or bad company.

Of course, similar scenarios play out in many people's lives, yet do not provoke speech changes. It is not possible to state definitively why for Paula speech became the focus of symptoms rather than myriad other ways in which issues might have manifested themselves. There is evidence that in functional disorders changes often echo some condition the person has already experienced – a sore throat, dental or maxillofacial injury, a choking episode (Baker et al., 2021; Espay et al., 2018).

Speculatively, this highlights a feasible factor. Paula already experienced speech changes with her hemiplegic migraines, how that felt for her, but, probably equally importantly, what responses this elicited from others. The semantic differential and impact questionnaires showed that Paula had a positive view of herself, but she could not fathom why people treated her so disparagingly. This undermined her positive beliefs, confidence and fostered depression and doubts. With the speech changes, Paula felt she now had a reason why people never believed or valued her opinions, talked down at her and why she felt 'inadequate' – she could hide behind speech difficulties to explain and excuse her behaviour and feelings, and as she had discovered, they proved a way of gaining attention.

Therapy

Two weeks following formal assessment, intervention commenced by discussing with Paula and her family how and why the diagnosis had been made, using assessment audio recordings to explain the positive, rule-in features of functional disorder and the implications of these for treatment options. Starting four weeks later she attended ten hours (10 × one hour/week) of cognitive behavioural therapy (CBT) (Birdsey & Millar, 2020; Gutkin, McLean, Brown, & Kanaan, 2020), reflecting on how/why speech played a role in the overall picture, understanding her reactions to others, and formulating coping strategies that avoided negative evaluation of herself instead of exploiting speech changes for temporary defence and/or gain. CBT sought positive strategies to assert and value herself and her work. Long-term plans explored advancing her career.

Initial speech work ran parallel to the CBT (3 × one hour/week). We did not target specific speech-motor parameters because these were not per se impaired. Work did entail exercises on minimal pair sound contrasts, loudness, prosody and word finding, aiming to reassure her they were not broken, and, crucially, to demonstrate she did have voluntary control over them. Follow-up speech sessions (3 × one hour/week) after CBT rehearsed strategies in for her gradually more challenging environments that would guarantee intelligibility when she felt she was going to relapse. These sessions also explored with her family how to support Paula in the positive communication strategies she had chosen.

With regained voice–speech status and confidence communicating work became positive again. She persuaded her employer to support further education. Within two years she successfully applied to study business and management at university.

Conclusions

Paula's case emphasises the importance, as ever, of careful history taking, within a non-threatening, trusting therapeutic relationship and that sometimes full facts may take a while to emerge. It stresses the importance of cross-checking details across all agencies and understanding the client and family views. It highlights the necessity of careful evaluation of data, not accepting a suspected diagnosis just because some perceived changes conformed to pre-expectations. Diagnostic decisions must stand up to fine, triangulated scrutiny. Regular reappraisal should confirm one is on the right path. Having imaging reports earlier probably would have hastened a functional diagnosis, but examination of Paula's speech patterns argued for this even before scan evidence availability.

Paula's case also illustrates the complex interrelationship between neurological/physical and psychological factors in functional disorders and that pathways to change start with the individual's beliefs about their condition and the position it holds in their life. The case showed that functional speech disorders can be successfully managed.

References

Assal, F., Laganaro, M., Remund, C. D., & Paquier, C. R. (2012). Progressive crossed-apraxia of speech as a first manifestation of a probable corticobasal degeneration. *Behavioural Neurology, 25*(4), 285–289. doi:10.3233/ben-2012-110219

Atkinson-Clement, C., Letanneux, A., Bailie, G., Cuartero, M.-C., Veron-Delor, L., Robieux, C., . . . Pinto, S. (2019). Psychosocial impact of dysarthria: The patient-reported outcome as part of the clinical management. *Neurodegenerative Diseases, 19*(1), 12–21. doi:10.1159/000499627

Baddeley, A., Emslie, H., & Nimmo-Smith, I. (1992). *Speed and Capacity of Language Processing Test (SCOLP)*. Oxford: PsychCorp.

Baker, J., Barnett, C., Cavalli, L., Dietrich, M., Dixon, L., Duffy, J. R., . . . McWhirter, L. (2021). Management of functional communication, swallowing, cough, and related disorders: Consensus recommendations for speech and language therapy. *Journal of Neurology Neurosurgery and Psychiatry*, 1–14. doi:10.1136/jnnp-2021-326767

Birdsey, N., & Millar, J. F. A. (2020). Cognitive behavioral therapy for foreign accent syndrome: A single-case experimental design. *Clinical Case Studies, 19*(5), 321–338. doi:10.1177/1534650120936771

Chung, D. S., Wettroth, C., Hallett, M., & Maurer, C. W. (2018). Functional speech and voice disorders: Case series and literature review. *Movement Disorders Clinical Practice, 5*(3), 312–316. doi:10.1002/mdc3.12609

DeBodt, M. S., Wuyts, F. L., VandeHeyning, P. H., & Croux, C. (1997). Test-retest study of the GRBAS scale: Influence of experience and professional background on perceptual rating of voice quality. *Journal of Voice, 11*(1), 74–80. ISI>://A1997WM86100009

Espay, A. J., Aybek, S., Carson, A., Edwards, M. J., Goldstein, L. H., Hallett, M., . . . Morgante, F. (2018). Current concepts in diagnosis and treatment of functional neurological disorders. *JAMA Neurology, 75*(9), 1132–1141. doi:10.1001/jamaneurol.2018.1264

Fernandes, P. M., Whiteley, W. N., Hart, S. R., & Al-Shahi Salman, R. (2013). Strokes: Mimics and chameleons. *Practical Neurology, 13*(1), 21–28. doi:10.1136/practneurol-2012-000465

Goodglass, H., & Kaplan, E. (2001). *Boston diagnostic aphasia examination*. Austin: Pro-Ed.

Gutkin, M., McLean, L., Brown, R., & Kanaan, R. A. (2020). Systematic review of psychotherapy for adults with functional neurological disorder. *Journal of Neurology, Neurosurgery, Psychiatry*. doi:10.1136/jnnp-2019-321926

Kaplan, E., Goodglass, H., & Weintraub, S. (2001). *Boston naming test:* Austin. Texas: Pro-Ed.

Marien, P., Paghera, B., De Deyn, P. P., & Vignolo, L. A. (2004). Adult crossed aphasia in dextrals revisited. *Cortex, 40*(1), 41–74. ISI>://000220483000006

McWhirter, L., Miller, N., Campbell, C., Hoeritzauer, I., Lawton, A., Carson, A., & Stone, J. (2019). Understanding foreign accent syndrome. *Journal of Neurology, Neurosurgery & Psychiatry*. doi:10.1136/jnnp-2018-319842

Mendez, M. F. (2018). Non-neurogenic language disorders: A preliminary classification. *Psychosomatics, 59*(1), 28–35. Retrieved from ISI://WOS:000418715900003

Miller, N. (2017). Communication changes in Parkinson's disease. *Practical Neurology, 17*(4), 266–274. doi:10.1136/practneurol-2017-001635

Miller, N., Nath, U., Noble, E., & Burn, D. (2017). Utility and accuracy of perceptual voice and speech distinctions in the diagnosis of Parkinson's disease, PSP and MSA-P. *Neurodegenerative Disease Management, 7*(3), 191–203. doi:10.2217/nmt-2017-0005

Miller, N., Noble, E., Jones, D., Allcock, L., & Burn, D. J. (2008). How do I sound to me? Perceived changes in communication in Parkinson's disease. *Clinical Rehabilitation, 22*(1), 14–22. doi:10.1177/0269215507079096

Miller, N., & Wambaugh, J. (2021). Apraxia of speech: Nature, assessment, treatment. In I. Papathanasiou & P. Coppens (Eds.), *Aphasia and related neurogenic communication disorders* (3rd ed., pp. 603–640). Boston, MA: Jones & Bartlett.

Montembeault, M., Brambati, S. M., Gorno-Tempini, M. L., & Migliaccio, R. (2018). Clinical, anatomical, and pathological features in the three variants of primary progressive aphasia: A review. *Frontiers in Neurology, 9*. doi:10.3389/fneur.2018.00692

Nadarajan, V., Perry, R. J., Johnson, J., & Werring, D. J. (2014). Transient ischaemic attacks: Mimics and chameleons. *Practical Neurology, 14*(1), 23–31. doi:10.1136/practneurol-2013-000782

Reilly, J., & Fisher, J. L. (2012). Sherlock Holmes and the strange case of the missing attribution: A historical note on "the Grandfather Passage". *Journal of Speech Language & Hearing Research, 55*(1), 84–88. doi:10.1044/1092-4388(2011/11-0158)

Romö, N., Miller, N., & Cardoso, A. (2021). Segmental diagnostics of neurogenic and functional foreign accent syndrome. *J Neurolinguistics, 58*. doi: https://doi.org/10.1016/j.jneuroling.2020.100983

Ryalls, J., & Miller, N. (2014). *Foreign accent syndromes: The stories people have to tell.* New York and Oxford: Guilford Press.

Takakura, Y., Otsuki, M., Sakai, S., Tajima, Y., Mito, Y., Ogata, A., . . . Nakagawa, Y. (2019). Sub-classification of apraxia of speech in patients with cerebrovascular and neurodegenerative diseases. *Brain Cognition, 130*, 1–10. doi: https://doi.org/10.1016/j.bandc.2018.11.005

Walshe, M., Peach, R., & Miller, N. (2009). Dysarthria impact profile: Development of a scale to measure the psychosocial impact of acquired dysarthria. *International Journal of Language & Communication Disorders, 44*(5), 693–715.

Whiteside, D. M., Kealey, T., Semla, M., Luu, H., Rice, L., Basso, M. R., & Roper, B. (2016). Verbal fluency: Language or executive function measure? *Applied Neuropsychology: Adult, 23*(1), 29–34. doi:10.1080/23279095.2015.1004574

Chapter 3

Dysarthria associated with hypoglossal nerve palsy and COVID-19

Irene Battel and Margaret Walshe

Introduction

This case report describes dysarthria due to bilateral hypoglossal nerve palsy. This cranial nerve (CNXII) is the motor supply to all the intrinsic and extrinsic muscles of the ipsilateral tongue, except palatoglossus. Subsequently, injuries to this nerve have the potential to significantly impact on a person's articulation and swallow function. RF, the focus of this case report, had COVID-19 resulting in dysarthria associated with CNXII injury. It is unclear whether dysarthria associated with CNXII paralysis arose as a result of neurological complications associated with COVID-19 or whether this dysarthria is linked to medical interventions such as intubation, proning and prolonged intensive care unit (ICU) stay and/or pharmaceutical management. In this chapter, we describe dysarthria arising from this isolated cranial nerve impairment and discuss the principles underlying the intervention approach used. The importance of telepractice in the delivery of treatment during a global pandemic is also emphasised.

Case report: RF

RF is a 42-year-old man who at the end of February 2020 presented to the emergency department of the local hospital in Italy with hyposmia, hypogeusia, respiratory difficulties and high fever, which did not respond to a generic antibiotic (amoxicillin). On day 5 of experiencing high fever, RF developed severe dyspnoea and he was admitted as an inpatient to the respiratory/pneumological department of the hospital. A COVID-19 swab test was positive. RF was healthy and physically active with no previous medical history prior to COVID-19 apart from mild bronchial asthma. He was isolated and commenced azithromycin and chloroquine therapy and received non-invasive ventilation using AIRVO™. AIRVO™ is typically used in the treatment of patients who are spontaneously breathing but would benefit from receiving high flow warmed and humidified respiratory gases.

DOI: 10.4324/9781003172536-3

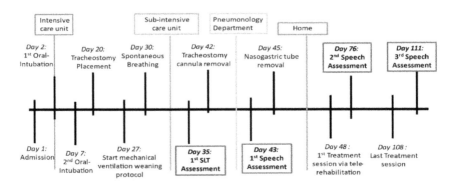

Figure 3.1 Timeline of the interventions carried out from hospitalisation to recovery

On the following day, RF developed further respiratory difficulties (oxygen saturation levels of 89–90%, low blood oxygen pressure PaO_2 = 57 mm Hg on gas analysis). He was transferred to the ICU. There, he was orally intubated for mechanical ventilation and sedated using the following medications: propofol, midazolam, remifentanil, neuromuscular block with curare and treated with remdesivir. He was proned according to the hospital's prone positioning protocol (six hours prone and six hours supine position). He was unable to feed orally due to sedation, and a nasogastric tube (NG) was sited. After a week in ICU, the first attempt of oral-tracheal extubation failed, RF had a desaturation crisis and he was orally re-intubated in order to be ventilated. Due to the difficulties with ventilation, the medical team decided to perform a tracheostomy and placed a Shiley™ size 8 tracheostomy cuffed tube.

After a week of mechanical ventilation with tracheostomy, blood gas analysis showed an improvement and RF started the weaning protocol from mechanical ventilation. When he was able to breathe independently without mechanical ventilation, he was transferred to a high-dependency unit (HDU). At this point, RF was referred to the speech and language therapist (SLT). She carried out a communication and swallowing assessment, and the decannulation protocol for the tracheostomy tube was initiated.

Neurological and neurophysiological examinations were carried out when RF was in the respiratory/pneumonology department, and the tracheostomy cannula was removed (Figure 3.1).

Electromyography (EMG) showed positive sharp waves within the genioglossus muscle suggesting an innervation deficit for CNXII. Magnetic resonance imaging found no evidence of cortical or brainstem lesions.

Clinical findings

The first speech and language assessment in the HDU revealed severe anarthria. RF was able to respond to closed-ended questions (YES/NO) using

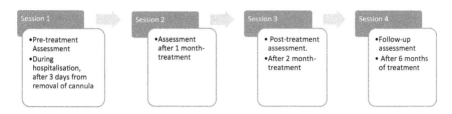

Figure 3.2 Timeline of speech and voice assessment

head movements. He communicated via written text, and he felt anxious about this inability to speak.

RF was hospitalised for 46 days (Figure 3.1). The first assessment conducted by the SLT was carried out when RF was able to self-ventilate on the 35th day of hospitalisation. This assessment focused on swallowing and respiratory function in order to facilitate the tracheostomy weaning process. On the 42nd day, the tracheostomy cannula was removed; the next day NG tube was also removed, and this facilitated discharge from the hospital.

Diagnostic assessment

The assessment protocol included an orofacial examination, a voice assessment, a drooling assessment and a dysarthria assessment. Assessments over the period of intervention were conducted at four time points: (1) pre-treatment, (2) after one-month of treatment, (3) post-treatment after two months and (4) follow-up assessment after six months (Figure 3.2).

Speech and voice assessment – session 1

Oro-motor examination: This included a cranial nerve assessment, completed using the validated I&I test assessment protocol (Koch et al., 2015). This revealed the following: severe bilateral CNXII palsy resulting in an absence of movements (lateralisation, elevation and protrusion) in the anterior two-thirds of the tongue. Muscle tone was noted to be flaccid. There was no evidence of sensory deficits. This was anticipated given that sensation of the tongue is supplied by the trigeminal (CNV), facial (CNVII) and glossopharyngeal (CNIX) nerves. There was a lot of saliva present in the oral cavity and RF presented with anterior drooling caused by difficulties managing and collecting secretions and saliva in the oral cavity, but this saliva was retained in the oral cavity. The Drooling Frequency and Drooling Severity Rating Scale (Thomas-Stonell & Greenberg, 1988) indicated mild drooling causing wet lips. Mild deficit of the oculomotor nerve (CNIII) resulting in a ptosis of the right eye was present. Motor and sensory functions of the other cranial nerves were not compromised.

Voice assessment: Laryngeal examination involved an instrumental fiber-optic endoscopic evaluation. Whilst this assessment was conducted for the purposes of examining swallowing safety at the pharyngeal and laryngeal levels, it also provided valuable information on laryngeal motility, which was described as normal. There was no impairment with adduction and abduction of the vocal folds. Oedema in the arytenoid mucosa was noted with laryngeal granulation above and beneath the vocal folds. Tissue granulation develops in response to irritation or injury. In this case, it was hypothesised that it was caused by the oral-tracheal intubation in ICU.

The SLT completed the Grade, Roughness, Breathiness, Asthenia, Strain scale (GRBAS) (Hirano, 1981), which revealed mild dysphonia (Grade: 2, Roughness: 2, Breathiness: 2, Asthenia: 3, Strain: 3). Nevertheless, due to COVID-19 infection control and protective measures, RF's voice was not recorded.

Dysarthria assessment: Dysarthria assessment was carried out using the Italian Robertson dysarthria profile (De Biagi, Frigo, Andrea, Sara, & Berta, 2018) (Table 3.1). Results indicated a severe deficit in all the subscales.

Quality of life: Quality of life was assessed using the Quality of Life related to Dysarthria (QOL-DyS) questionnaire (Piacentini, Zuin, Cattaneo, & Schindler, 2011), which comprises seven domains. The most impaired domains were perceived speech characteristics, situational difficulties, compensatory strategy and perceived reaction. Performance on all the subscales showed compromise, indicating severe impairment (total score: 142/160). RF reported that he was anxious about his future and worried that his work as a dentist could be affected by the speech impairment. Following this assessment, RF commenced an intervention programme at his home via telepractice. The programme lasted for two months and is detailed in the next section.

Intervention programme

Treatment incorporated the following motor learning and neuroplasticity principles: (1) task-specific practice, (2) use and improve it, (3) feedback, (4) repetition matters, (5) intensity matters and (6) time matters (Kleim & Jones, 2008; Maas et al., 2008; Roller, 2012) (Table 3.2). Treatment was scheduled for one hour per day, five days a week for eight weeks, using the Google Meet video platform (https://meet.google.com).

Week 1: The treatment included passive tongue manipulation to increase the active movement of the tongue. The passive manipulation of the

Table 3.1 Results of the Italian Robertson Dysarthria Profile at the first assessment session

Respiration and phonation	Ability to sustain /s/	12 seconds
	Shallow respiration and deficit in pneumo-phono articulatory coordination.	
	Maximum phonation duration /a/	12 seconds
	Breathlessness	
	Severe hypophonia, difficulty saying three consecutive words aloud.	
Diadochokinetic	Normal for the task /oo-ee/ and /pa-pa/	
	Severe impaired for /ka-la/ and /puh-tuh-kuh/	
Oral-facial motility	Absence of any tongue movements (protrusion, lateralisation and elevation).	
	Hypotonia of the tongue	
	Motility of facial muscles was normal, but ptosis was present.	
Articulation	Severe impairment of articulation and co-articulation of the following phonemes: dental, alveolar, post-alveolar, affricate alveolar, retroflex, palatal and velar consonants.	
	No difficulty on labial sounds /p/,b/.	
Intelligibility	Intelligibility was 15% at word level, caused by imprecise oral articulation. Intelligibility at sentence level was 30%.	
	Using the Yorkston Rating of Dysarthria Severity Scale (Donovan et al., 2008), RF was at Stage 4: Natural speech supplemented by augmentative techniques: Natural speech alone is no longer functional. Frequent communication breakdowns. Severe dysarthria with minimal speech intelligibility.	
Prosody	No prosodic impairments were noted. However, intonation and the rhythm of the spontaneous speech were affected by articulation and phonation difficulties.	

tongue was hypothesised to play a role in facilitating tongue movements, and it was combined with visual feedback through using a mirror. Action observation training is recognised to increase motor performance mainly for limb paralysis in stroke rehabilitation (Mizuguchi & Kanosue, 2017; Sarasso, Gemma, Agosta, Filippi, & Gatti, 2015; Zhang et al., 2019). In addition, RF monitored the contraction of his neck muscles during lingual tasks: a maladaptive behaviour noted initially. It is likely that these muscles were activated in order to compensate for the absence of tongue movements. Maladaptive behaviours were thus discouraged (Table 3.3).

Table 3.2 Description of the neuroplasticity and motor learning principles applied to the treatment

Principle	Description	Application
Task-specific practice	Motor learning occurs when training is purposeful and related to the skills to be acquired.	The speech treatment was customised accordingly with tasks specifically focused on tongue movement and articulation.
Use and improve it	Increasing competence in terms of efficiency or accuracy leads to neural modification and improvements.	RF was encouraged to speak as much as possible to improve articulation.
Feedback	Providing signals to increase awareness of ongoing movements in order to accomplish the correct performance.	A mirror was used by RF for visual feedback for tongue movements, and audio recording was also used to help auditory self-mownitoring of articulation. Verbal feedback on performance was provided within sessions.
Repetition matters	Consistent practice is fundamental for learning and maintaining the targeted function.	The speech treatment involved several repetition of the tongue movements and articulation tasks.
Intensity matters	Concentrated exercise with high intensity is important.	The scheduled speech treatment was intense, one hour a day, five days a week, for eight weeks. RF also completed exercises independently.
Time matters	The timing of intervention and the duration of the intervention is known to influence recovery.	Intervention started at the early stages of recovery from COVID-19. This was important also for psychological support and to prevent maladaptive behaviours.
Salience	Therapy must be meaningful to the person in order to cause change.	RF reported that the lingual deficit was severe and disabling. He considered this speech rehabilitation fundamental to his ability to return to his work and social life.

Weeks 2–4: In this treatment period, the focus was on skill rather than strength exercises for the tongue, as RF gained more control over lingual movements. As soon as RF started to achieve some tongue movements, passive exercises were discontinued to foster active lingual movements (recruitment). These skill exercises aimed to achieve fine control of the tongue during verbal tasks in order to increase articulation and coarticulation during speech (week 4) (Table 3.3).

Speech and voice assessment – session 2

This assessment was carried out after one month of treatment, and it revealed a complete recovery of voice and drooling symptoms. Although articulation had improved with increased tongue movements, speech remained dysarthric (Table 3.4).

Oro-motor examination: The cranial nerve assessment 'I&I test' (Koch et al., 2015) was repeated and showed an improvement only for the CNXII from severe to mild palsy. Tongue protrusion to the inferior lip was possible, although RM could not reach maximum extension. Lateralisation outside and inside the mouth on the right side was possible, although there were tremors during the performance of maximum extension. Lateralisation outside the mouth on the left side was compromised, but some movements of the tip of the tongue were possible inside the mouth. Lateralisation increased with the mouth closed. Elevation inside the oral cavity was not possible with mouth open; nevertheless, RF could reach the alveolar palatal area with the mouth open. The mild deficit of the oculomotor nerve (CNIII) remained stable with a ptosis of the right eye.

Voice assessment: The GRBAS scale (Hirano, 1981) showed the absence of dysphonia now.

Dysarthria assessment: The Italian Robertson dysarthria profile (De Biagi et al., 2018) showed a slight improvement in all subscales (Table 3.4)

Drooling assessment: The Drooling Frequency and Drooling Severity Rating Scale (Thomas-Stonell & Greenberg, 1988) indicated the absence of drooling.

Quality of Life: The QOL-DyS (Piacentini et al., 2011) showed overall quality of life changes from severe (total score: 142/160) to mild (total score: 63/160). The most impaired domains remained perceived speech characteristics (score: 27/40) and situational difficulties (24/40). Nevertheless, RM continued to be worried about his future and work, which could be affected by his speech impairment.

Table 3.3 Intervention programme

	Type of exercises	Instructions	Repetition	Feedback	Aims	Principles
Week 1	Active exercise	Try to protrude/lateralise the tongue. (If you cannot do this, try to imagine the movement) Try not to contract the supplementary neck muscles, during tasks	5 × 10 times	Mirror Verbal feedback from SLT	Stimulation active tongue movement	Task-specific Use and improve it Repetition Intensity matter Time matters
	Passive exercise	Tongue manipulation in protrusion and lateralisation position.				
	Voice exercise	Humming voice exercise and lip buzzing and trill exercises	3 × 10 times		Increase voice quality	
Week 2–3	Active exercise	Try to touch the inferior dental arch with tip of the tongue Tongue lateralisation	10 × 5 (week 1) 10 × 8 (week 2)	Mirror		Task-specific Use and improve it Repetition Intensity matter Time matters Salience

Week 4	Active exercise	During lateralisation and protrusion, hold max extension for 5 seconds	Hold 10 s × 20		Stimulation of active tongue movement
		Tongue lateralisation Tongue protrusion Try to touch the palate with the tongue and the mouth open	10 times × 10		
		During lateralisation and protrusion, hold max extension	Hold 10 s × 20	Proprioception	
		Move one small candy from one side to the other of oral cavity			
	Articulation exercises	Read a list of words containing cluster of alveolar, retroflex consonants		Audio recording	Increase fine movements of the tongue during verbal production
Week 1–4	Voice exercise	Humming voice exercise and lip buzzing and trill	5 × 10 times		Increase voice quality

Speech and voice assessment – session 2

(Continued)

Table 3.3 Continued

	Type of exercises	Instructions	Repetition	Feedback	Aims	Principles
Week 5–7	Active exercise	Tongue lateralisation, protrusion and elevation	10 × 10 times	Mirror	Stimulation of active tongue movement	Task-specific Use and improve it Repetition Intensity matter Time matters Salience
		Hold max extension Paying attention at the accuracy of the movement				
		Move one small candy within the oral cavity	5 × 10 times	Proprioception	Increase lingual fine movements and Intelligibility	
	Articulation exercises	Increase articulation during reading tasks and spontaneous speech	10 minutes	Audio recording		
Week 8	Articulation and coarticulation exercises	Increase articulation during reading tasks and spontaneous speech	10 minutes	Audio recording	Increase Intelligibility	

Post-treatment speech and voice assessment – session 3

Table 3.4 Results of the Italian Robertson dysarthria profile at the second assessment session

Respiration and phonation	Ability to sustain /s/	15 seconds
	Maximum phonation duration /a/	12 seconds
	Improved respiratory-voice coordination.	
	No hypophonia.	
Diadochokinetic	Normal /oo-ee/ and /pa-pa/	
	Severe impaired for /ka-la/	
Oral-facial motility	Difficulties during protrusion, lateralisation of the tongue.	
	No elevation of the tongue with the mouth open, mild elevation with the closed mouth.	
	Motility of facial muscles was normal, but ptosis remained stable and present.	
Articulation	Mild difficulties of articulation and co-articulation of the following phonemes: post-alveolar, retroflex; affricate alveolar mostly in clusters of 2–3 consonants.	
	No deficit for articulation of other consonants or hypernasality.	
Intelligibility	Intelligibility was at 45% at the sentence level.	
	Using the Yorkston Rating of Dysarthria Severity scale (Donovan et al., 2008), RF was now at Stage 2: *Obvious speech disorder with intelligible speech.*	
Prosody	No significant prosodic deficit evident.	

Intervention programme

Weeks 4–8: It is argued that non-speech oro-motor exercises do not improve articulation and intelligibility of speech (Maas et al., 2008; Mitchell, Bowen, Tyson, Butterfint, & Conroy, 2017; Park, Theodoros, Finch, & Cardell, 2016), but RF needed to achieve some movements and voluntary control of his tongue. As soon as this movement was achieved, intervention focused on articulation incorporating the principles of 'use it and improve it' – working directly on articulation to improve articulation (Table 3.3).

Thereafter, RF underwent a third speech assessment at the hospital, which confirmed that the treatment goals for communication were achieved. These were to improve tongue function for speech and to increase speech intelligibility and comprehensibility.

Speech and voice assessment – session 3

The third assessment was completed after two months of treatment. RF showed no signs of speech impairment; the articulation and motility of the tongue were normal.

> *Neurophysiologic examination:* Repeat EMG assessment revealed a complete recovery of innervation of the genioglossus muscle.
>
> *Oro-motor examination:* The cranial nerve assessment using the 'I&I test' (Koch et al., 2015) revealed no signs of hypoglossal nerve deficit. The motility of tongue was normal but remaining mild deficit of the oculomotor nerve (CNIII) showing a ptosis of the right eye.
>
> *Dysarthria assessment:* The Italian Robertson dysarthria profile (De Biagi et al., 2018) showed no signs of dysarthria in any of the subscales. The respiration and phonation sub-scale showed normal scores (ability to sustain /s/: 16 seconds; maximum phonation duration /a/: 14 seconds). Intelligibility was normal at both word and sentence levels (Stage 1 of the Yorkston Rating of Dysarthria Severity scale: No detectable speech problem (Donovan et al., 2008).
>
> *Quality of Life:* Quality of life, assessed using QOL-DyS (Piacentini et al., 2011), was normal. The total score was 10/160, which revealed good quality of life.

Speech and voice assessment – session 4

A follow-up assessment was carried out after six months from the third assessment to check maintenance of function, and RF had maintained function. He had returned to his baseline pre-COVID-19 status and reported that he had resumed normal activities and he did not perceive any difficulties during speaking.

Nevertheless, the ptosis of the right eye did not improve, although it was mild. RF reported that this oculo-motor deficit worsened when he was tired.

Discussion

This case report describes the management of a motor speech disorder as a consequence of COVID-19. The cause of dysarthria was attributed to CNXII. Lesions of hypoglossal nerve during manoeuvring for oral intubation have been described in several studies (Cinar, Seven, Cinar, & Turgut, 2005; De Luca et al., 2020; Decavel, Petit, & Tatu, 2020; Dziewas & Lüdemann, 2002; Lykoudis & Seretis, 2012; Shah, Barnes, Spiekerman, & Bollag, 2015). Hypoglossal nerve damage may also occur as a result of proning. Decavel et al. describe a patient with COVID-19 who required prolonged prone-position ventilation with lateral flexion of the head (Decavel et al., 2020). In a post-acute care unit, this patient presented with left hypoglossal nerve paralysis and left soft palate weakness along with complete paralysis of the left vocal cord in the abducted position. The authors concluded that the prone-position ventilation could be the main aetiological factor; nevertheless, they did not report about intervention and whether the patient recovered.

The question is whether this hypoglossal nerve palsy could spontaneously recover without intervention. Shah et al., in a review of the literature on hypoglossal nerve palsy, found that complete recovery of the CNXII was not achieved in 10 of 25 studies (Shah et al., 2015). Recently, due to the increased need for mechanical ventilation in patients with COVID-19, there is an increase in the number of studies, which describe the side effects of oral intubation in swallowing, voice and speech (Brodsky & Gilbert, 2020; Frajkova, Tedla, Tedlova, Suchankova, & Geneid, 2020; Schindler et al., 2020; Simpson & Robinson, 2020). Similar to RF, two studies report unilateral hypoglossal palsy in patients with COVID-19 (Costa Martins, Branco Ribeiro, Jesus Pereira, Mestre, & Rios, 2020; Decavel et al., 2020). Decavel et al. describe unilateral lower cranial neuropathy following prolonged intubation in a patient with COVID-19 as mentioned earlier, and Costa Martins et al. describe a patient with unilateral palsy who was discharged from the hospital on Day 43 post-admission showing a significant clinical improvement after treatment by SLT, although 'maintaining some degree of right deviation and hemi-atrophy of the tongue' (Costa Martins et al., 2020). Nevertheless, in the Costa Martins et al. study, the patient did not continue speech treatment after hospitalisation; he was monitored only at ambulatory follow-up, and complete recovery of tongue function was not reported.

Key messages

There are a number of key points to consider in this case report. First, it is hypothesised that the intensity of treatment incorporating the principles of motor learning and neural plasticity played a role in the recovery of RF's tongue function and dysarthria. It is worth noting that the ptosis remained an issue and did not mirror the recovery of speech. Second, the role of non-speech oro-motor exercises in improving speech intelligibility in dysarthria is subject to debate (Mackenzie, Muir, Allen, & Jensen, 2014). In this case report, RF had minimal tongue movement and some lingual exercises were required not just for speech but also for swallowing. As his tongue movements increased, his swallowing also improved, thus further enhancing tongue movement. The relationship between improvement in tongue function and improvement in speech is not linear, but perhaps in the presence of an isolated hypoglossal nerve lesion, people, such as RF, may gain some benefits from non-speech oro-motor exercises. Third, in this case report, telepractice during this global pandemic facilitated implementation of an intensive customised treatment for RF at home. Attendance at the hospital for rehabilitation was not possible due to restrictions on outpatient clinics. In addition to these restrictions during the COVID-19 pandemic, RF continued to have respiratory difficulties post-hospital discharge. He needed to stop and sit after 8–10 minutes of walking. It is established that COVID-19 is associated with chronic fatigue (Varatharaj et al., 2020). The delivery of the intervention via telepractice meant that RF could receive intensive therapy that otherwise would not be possible. RF gives his perspective in the next and final section.

Patient perspective

When they removed my tracheostomy tube, I realized that I could no longer speak. The tongue didn't move and my voice was different. From that period, I remember the loneliness, anxiety and fear that I was no longer able to speak and work as a dentist, but at the same time I had a desire to go home. After almost 2 months of hospitalization, I wanted to return to my normal life, although I did not want to interrupt the SLT's treatment. In addition, I was very weak, I had lost 20 kg and was unable to continue the outpatient treatment. So, the telepractice was essential for me.

Regarding the treatment, the first few weeks were very frustrating, because the movements of the tongue were minimal, even though I tried to move it as hard as I could. Working with the mirror helped me to realize how far I could move my tongue and make the movements better. After the first month of treatment, I was able to actively move my tongue, although the movements were not precise and I was unable to lateralize it to the left and raise it. Articulation improved more and more week by week as evidenced by the various interviews I did on television and in the news. The most difficult sound was /r/, which did not vibrate. I felt like I was speaking like a foreigner. Towards the middle of July, I realized that I was 'healed' because nobody noticed how I spoke, I spoke as before.

References

Brodsky, M. B., & Gilbert, R. J. (2020). The long-term effects of COVID-19 on dysphagia evaluation and treatment. *Archives of Physical Medicine and Rehabilitation*, 101(9), 1662–1664.

Cinar, S. O., Seven, H., Cinar, U., & Turgut, S. (2005). Isolated bilateral paralysis of the hypoglossal and recurrent laryngeal nerves (bilateral Tapia's syndrome) after transoral intubation for general anesthesia. *Acta Anaesthesiologica Scandinavica*, 49(1), 98–99.

Costa Martins, D., Branco Ribeiro, S., Jesus Pereira, I., Mestre, S., & Rios, J. (2020). Unilateral hypoglossal nerve palsy as a COVID-19 sequel. *American Journal of Physical Medicine & Rehabilitation*, 99(12), 1096–1098.

De Biagi, F., Frigo, A., Andrea, T., Sara, N., & Berta, G. (2018). Italian validation of a test to assess dysarthria in neurologic patients: A cross-sectional pilot study. *Otolaryngology (Sunnyvale)*, 8(1), 343–349.

De Luca, P., Cavaliere, M., Scarpa, A., Savignano, L., Cassandro, E., Cassandro, C., & Iemma, M. (2020). Rehabilitation protocol for unilateral laryngeal and lingual paralysis (Tapia syndrome): Comment about "a challenging case of Tapia syndrome after total thyroidectomy" by Ildem Deveci, Mehmet Surmeli, and Reyhan Surmeli. *Ear, Nose & Throat Journal*. 10.

Decavel, P., Petit, C., & Tatu, L. (2020). Tapia syndrome at the time of the COVID-19 pandemic: Lower cranial neuropathy following prolonged intubation. *Neurology*, 95(7), 312–313.

Donovan, N. J., Kendall, D. L., Young, M. E., & Rosenbek, J. C. (2008). The communicative effectiveness survey: Preliminary evidence of construct validity. *American Journal of Speech-Language Pathology*, 17(4), 335–347.

Dziewas, R., & Lüdemann, P. (2002). Hypoglossal nerve palsy as complication of oral intubation, bronchoscopy and use of the laryngeal mask airway. *European Journal of Neurology*, 47(4), 239–243.

Frajkova, Z., Tedla, M., Tedlova, E., Suchankova, M., & Geneid, A. (2020). Postintubation dysphagia during COVID-19 outbreak-contemporary review. *Dysphagia*, 35(4), 549–557.

Hirano, M. (1981). *Clinical Examination of Voice*. Springer-Verlag, New York.

Kleim, J. A., & Jones, T. A. (2008). Principles of experience-dependent neural plasticity: Implications for rehabilitation after brain damage. *Journal of Speech, Language, and Hearing Research*, 51(1), S225–S239.

Koch, I., Ferrazzi, A., Busatto, C., Ventura, L., Palmer, K., Stritoni, P., . . . Battel, I. (2015). Cranial nerve examination for neurogenic dysphagia patients. *Journal of Patient Care*, 1(1).

Lykoudis, E. G., & Seretis, K. (2012). Tapia's syndrome: An unexpected but real complication of rhinoplasty: Case report and literature review. *Aesthetic Plastic Surgery*, 36(3), 557–559.

Maas, E., Robin, D. A., Austermann Hula, S. N., Freedman, S. E., Wulf, G., Ballard, K. J., & Schmidt, R. A. (2008). Principles of motor learning in treatment of motor speech disorders. *American Journal of Speech-Language Pathology*, 17(3), 277–298.

Mackenzie, C., Muir, M., Allen, C., & Jensen, A. (2014). Non-speech oro-motor exercises in post-stroke dysarthria intervention: A randomized feasibility trial. *International Journal of Language & Communication Disorders*, 49(5), 602–617.

Mitchell, C., Bowen, A., Tyson, S., Butterfint, Z., & Conroy, P. (2017). Interventions for dysarthria due to stroke and other adult-acquired, non-progressive brain injury. *Cochrane Database of Systematic Reviews*, 1(1), CD002088.

Mizuguchi, N., & Kanosue, K. (2017). Changes in brain activity during action observation and motor imagery: Their relationship with motor learning. *Progress in Brain Research*, 234, 189–204.

Park, S., Theodoros, D., Finch, E., & Cardell, E. (2016). Be clear: A new intensive speech treatment for adults with nonprogressive dysarthria. *American Journal of Speech-Language Pathology*, 25(1), 97–110.

Piacentini, V., Zuin, A., Cattaneo, D., & Schindler, A. (2011). Reliability and validity of an instrument to measure quality of life in the dysarthric speaker. *Folia Phoniatrica et Logopaedica*, 63(6), 289–295.

Roller, M. L. (2012). Control, motor learning, and neuroplasticity. *Neurological Rehabilitation*, 69.

Sarasso, E., Gemma, M., Agosta, F., Filippi, M., & Gatti, R. (2015). Action observation training to improve motor function recovery: A systematic review. *Archives of Physiotherapy*, 5(14).

Schindler, A., Baijens, L. W. J., Clave, P., Degen, B., Duchac, S., Dziewas, R., . . . Rommel, N. (2021). ESSD commentary on dysphagia management during COVID pandemia. *Dysphagia*, 36(4), 764–767.

Shah, A. C., Barnes, C., Spiekerman, C. F., & Bollag, L. A. (2015). Hypoglossal nerve palsy after airway management for general anesthesia: An analysis of 69 patients. *Anesthesia and Analgesia*, 120(1), 105–120.

Simpson, R., & Robinson, L. (2020). Rehabilitation following critical illness in people with COVID-19 infection. *American Journal of Physical Medicine & Rehabilitation*, 99(6), 470–474.

Thomas-Stonell, N., & Greenberg, J. (1988). Three treatment approaches and clinical factors in the reduction of drooling. *Dysphagia*, 3(2), 73–78.

Varatharaj, A., Thomas, N., Ellul, M. A., Davies, N., Pollak, T. A., Tenorio, E. L., . . . Coro-Nerve Study Group. (2020). Neurological and neuropsychiatric complications of COVID-19 in 153 patients: A UK-wide surveillance study. *Lancet Psychiatry*, 7(10), 875–882.

Zhang, B., Kan, L., Dong, A., Zhang, J., Bai, Z., Xie, Y., . . . Peng, Y. (2019). The effects of action observation training on improving upper limb motor functions in people with stroke: A systematic review and meta-analysis. *PLoS One*, 14(8), e0221166.

Chapter 4

Case report on speech treatment of a young adult with Down syndrome

Leslie Mahler

Introduction

Many neurological disorders of childhood can cause difficulty with speech, language or cognition that interfere with communication effectiveness. A neurological disorder can be present at birth or acquired shortly after birth whilst the child's nervous system is developing. Down syndrome (DS) is an example of a genetic disorder present at birth caused by an abnormality of chromosome 21. It results in an extra chromosome that interferes with normal growth and development. Down syndrome occurs in approximately 1 in 700 births in the United States (Parker et al., 2010). All children with DS experience cognitive delays, and many have deficits in language and motor speech control. Reduced speech intelligibility caused by dysarthria in people with DS can negatively impact communication effectiveness and social participation because it contributes to communication breakdowns (Kent & Vorperian, 2013). A research study by Jones, Crisp, Kuchibhatla, Mahler, Risoli, Jones, & Kishnani (2019) described the auditory-perceptual speech features of children with DS suggesting that distributed motor speech impairment associated with dysarthria could be addressed with treatment. Speech intelligibility in people with DS can improve between ages 4 and 16 but may still interfere with communication into adulthood (Wild, Vorperian, Kent, Bolt, & Austin, 2018). A case series study of perceptual and acoustic speech characteristics of people with DS included two adults ages 27 and 44 years. The results of those analyses revealed that the most frequently occurring deficits interfering with speech intelligibility were consonant errors, distorted vowels, breathy voice quality and reduced pitch variation (O'Leary, Lee, O'Toole, & Gibbon, 2020). Whilst these findings expand on the connection of DS with speech deficits, there is little evidence of the effects of motor speech treatment for people with DS at any age even though the negative influence of dysarthria on communication has been identified (Stoel-Gammon, 2001).

People with DS have an increased risk for medical conditions such as congenital heart defects and respiratory problems that can threaten longevity. However, these conditions are treatable, and the life expectancy for people

DOI: 10.4324/9781003172536-4

with DS has increased dramatically from an average life expectancy of 25 years of age in 1983 to 60 years of age in 2017 (National Down Syndrome Society, retrieved 20 December 2020). Many adults with DS are community dwelling for many years of their adult life with minimal available services to support them (Smith, 2001). Janet Carr, a clinical psychologist, began a longitudinal study in 1964 and published results when the participants were 30 years of age (Carr, 2000) and 50 years of age (Carr & Collins, 2018). The total sample size reduced from the original 54 participants over the years. Thirteen deaths occurred before 30 years of age and one shortly thereafter. Results from the study of 40, 30-year-old participants suggested that the post-school years of people with DS showed no significant decline or improvement in mental ability or self-care skills with the majority remaining in the care of their parents (Carr, 2000). The study of 27, 50-year-old participants found that 18% of the participants had experienced a significant decline in mental ability and either were suspected of having dementia or had confirmed dementia (Carr & Collins, 2018). Overall, the results of this longitudinal study suggest that there is a stable time in young adulthood during which people with DS might benefit from behavioural interventions. However, this is not a time when behavioural interventions are typically offered. A study by Docherty & Reid (2009) explored the values and beliefs of eight mothers of young adults with DS. The interviews revealed that mothers perceived one of their roles as supporting their children to transition to greater independence. Increased understandability of speech and improved speech naturalness could contribute to facilitating greater independence in adult life for people with DS supporting the goal of these parents.

Advances in health care have extended the lifespan of people with DS, yet services to support them as adults are minimal (Smith, 2001). A longer life expectancy means that health care providers, including speech-language pathologists, should consider the role of dysarthria treatment across the lifespan. To date, most research about the treatment of people with DS has focused on children under the age of 21 years. This case report will describe behavioural speech treatment administered to a young woman with DS who sought services to improve speech comprehensibility with the goal of increasing confidence for social participation and gaining greater independence.

Case report: DS

DS was 34 years old at the time of the study. She was born 13 weeks premature and diagnosed with DS at three days. She was hospitalised several times during her first year of life for underdevelopment and failure to thrive. A heart murmur was diagnosed at three months of age, and she was treated with mitral valve replacement and a pacemaker. No other significant medical history was reported. DS received early intervention services including speech-language pathology until three years of age. Her mother reported that she was delayed in her production of speech sounds and did not begin using single words until after three years of age. She continued to receive services for language and cognition whilst at school until age 21 but did not receive services for dysarthria. DS began attending an interactive day programme for adults with developmental disabilities after she left the public school system with the hope of developing skills to gain employment and increase social participation and independence. She was referred for speech-language pathology services to address these goals by improving speech understandability.

Clinical findings/diagnostic focus and assessment

DS demonstrated language and cognitive deficits as well as dysarthria, in her initial evaluation. She received a 76.2 Aphasia Quotient on the Western Aphasia Battery-Revised (Kertesz, 2006), and results of subtests of the Repeatable Battery for the Assessment of Neurological Status were 16/40 on list learning and naming five items in one minute on semantic fluency. DS's speech characteristics were consistent with a diagnosis of moderate flaccid dysarthria. Her speech included imprecise consonants, irregular vowels, decreased vocal intensity, an intermittent breathy vocal quality, reduced pitch variation and mild hypernasality. Speech sound errors consisted of consonant substitutions, medial and final consonant deletions and consonant blend simplifications. DS's speech intelligibility for single words was 62.67% at her initial evaluation. The Goldman Fristoe 2, Test of Articulation (Goldman & Fristoe, 2000) was administered to identify patterns of phoneme errors that could be targeted in treatment.

Equipment and recording procedures

Evaluation data were obtained in a sound-treated booth where DS received repeated measures of the dependent variables over four days under control conditions during the A phases of the study. A head-mounted microphone (Isomax B3 omnidirectional lavalier microphone, Countryman Associates, Redwood City, CA) was fitted to her head with a mouth-to-microphone distance of 8 cm to obtain an accurate speech signal (48-kHz sampling rate, 16-bit quantisation). This signal was relayed to a pre-amplifier (Universal audio 4110) to assure quality signal acquisition and then converted from an analog to a digital signal using a Fireface converter (model RME ADI-8 DSI). The digitised acoustic signal was recorded to a computer hard drive. A Level I sound level metre (Bruel & Kjaer 2239) was used to collect vocal intensity simultaneously during the speech recordings. Five listeners unfamiliar with DS listened to a recording of 50 phonetically balanced single words and were instructed to write the words that they heard. The total number of words accurately identified by the listeners was used to calculate percentage intelligibility scores. Listeners were blinded to the time of the recordings.

Therapeutic focus and assessment

Two distinct behavioural speech treatments to improve comprehensibility were administered in an A-B-A-Withdrawal-A-C-A single subject experimental design. Please refer to Figure 4.1 for a timeline of the evaluations and interventions. The first treatment focused on voice with the goal of increasing vocal intensity to levels congruent with DS's age and gender. The first treatment administered was LSVT LOUDâ, a behavioural voice treatment that incorporates principles of motor learning, which was originally developed for people with Parkinson's disease (Ramig, Halpern, Spielman, Fox, & Freeman, 2018; Randolph, Tierney, Mohr, & Chase, 1998). LSVT LOUD incorporates principles of motor learning such as intensity of practice with high repetitions of salient materials that is also relevant for treating people with DS who have impaired cognitive abilities. Research of LSVT LOUD outcomes has demonstrated a distributed impact of treatment to articulation even though only voice is directly targeted in treatment, which is one reason this treatment approach was chosen. A study by Sapir, Spielman, Ramig, Story, & Fox (2007) identified larger vowel space area following treatment, and Dromey, Ramig, & Johnson (1995) identified improved articulatory acoustics after treatment. LSVT LOUD was also chosen based on the specific speech characteristics of DS which included reduced intensity, a breathy voice quality and decreased pitch variation in addition to imprecise articulation. Research using LSVT LOUD in case studies of persons with a variety of dysarthria types has been previously demonstrated (Mahler & Jones, 2012; Mahler & Ramig, 2012; Mahler, Ramig, & Fox, 2015) further supporting the rationale for this treatment approach. LSVT LOUD uses high effort exercises to increase vocal loudness to a level that is within normal limits using healthy and efficient voice techniques. The first half of every session consisted of daily exercises that formed the foundation for teaching normal loudness in conversation.

The second round of treatment was undertaken at the completion of LSVT LOUD to address residual articulation deficits with the goal of further improving speech comprehensibility. Articulation treatment also used high effort exercises aimed to make phoneme production more precise. Both treatments incorporated principles of motor learning and were administered with the same dosage: four times a week for four weeks totalling 16 one-hour individual sessions each.

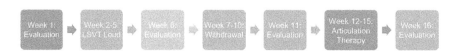

Figure 4.1 Timeline of evaluations and interventions

It has been proposed that incorporating motor learning principles such as intensity of practice with high repetitions of salient materials may be beneficial for motor speech disorders in general (Maas, Robin, Hula, Freedman, Wulf, Ballard, & Schmidt, 2008). The following items explain how motor learning principles were translated to both of DS's treatments.

- Practice amount: the dosage of treatment was four times a week for four weeks totalling 16 one-hour individual treatment sessions. There were multiple repetitions of each task within each treatment session providing consistent exercise throughout the 60-minute treatment sessions. Also, there were 28 days of homework and carryover tasks that included days when DS did not attend treatment.
- Practice distribution: daily tasks for each treatment were repeated multiple times in a small period of time and repeated across all treatment sessions.
- Practice variability: the majority of each treatment session consisted of using treatment targets in the context of real speech providing practice of the targets in variable authentic communication contexts.
- Attentional focus: there was an external focus on the acoustic signal rather than on specific articulatory or speech gestures, for two reasons. Improved intelligibility and speech naturalness were the goals for treatment and were measured by acoustic outcome variables. Second is that speech is a complex task and focusing on specifics of speech movement would increase the cognitive load for DS interfering with her ability to focus on the primary treatment target of vocal intensity or clear speech.
- Target complexity: the hierarchy allowed treatment task length and complexity to gradually increase over the course of treatment maximising the potential for carryover outside of the treatment environment.
- Feedback type and frequency: the type and frequency of feedback were carefully planned to facilitate generalisation of treatment targets. Feedback was based on the accuracy of the acoustic signal, and the amount of feedback was gradually decreased over the course of treatment for DS to learn the treatment targets and become independent with loudness and clear speech strategies.

Table 4.1 describes activities for LSVT LOUD, and Table 4.2 describes activities for articulation treatment.

Outcomes and follow-up

DS was motivated and fully participated throughout both treatments. Dependent variables used to assess her response to treatment included vocal intensity

Table 4.1 LSVT LOUD treatment tasks and aims during individual 60-minute sessions

	LSVT LOUD exercise	Aims
Daily Exercises	Sustained vowel phonation of /a/ for as long as possible with good voice quality (15 repetitions)	Improve vocal fold adduction and increase coordination of respiration and phonation for greater intensity of speech in conversation
	High- and low-pitch exercises; start at speaking fundamental frequency and then change pitch and hold for five seconds (15 repetitions)	Increase pitch range for greater frequency variation in conversation
	Read functional phrases that DS says every day (10 minutes)	Incorporate increased vocal intensity and pitch variation from the first two exercises in sentences that the person says every day
Hierarchy		
Week 1	Read words and phrases (30 minutes)	Use increased amplitude while reading words and sentences to manage cognitive demands of the task and focus on vocal intensity
Week 2	Read sentences and short answer conversation (30 minutes)	Use increased amplitude while reading sentences and during short answer conversation to incorporate increased vocal intensity
Week 3	Read short paragraphs and longer answer conversation (30 minutes)	Use increased amplitude during longer reading, structured dialogue and conversation to incorporate increased vocal intensity
Week 4	Conversation (30 minutes)	Use increased amplitude during structured dialogue and conversation to generalise increased vocal intensity in functional communication
Cue	Say that with **normal loudness**	Maintain the focus on vocal intensity
Homework	A subset of daily exercises and assignments based on DS's activities (20 minutes)	Carryover and generalisation of treatment targets outside of the clinical environment

measured by vocal sound pressure level (dB SPL), the acoustic correlate of loudness, during vowel prolongation, sentence reading, picture description and monologue. In addition, data on single-word intelligibility as judged by unfamiliar listeners were obtained. Lip and lingual strength measured by the

Table 4.2 Articulation treatment tasks and aims during individual 60-minute sessions

	Articulation exercise	Aims
Daily Exercises	IOPI lip and tongue tip exercises: one set of five repetitions each. IOPI bulb placement between anterior lips and between tongue blade and hard palate (5 minutes)	Provide a kinaesthetic reference for increased effort of articulation using the cue to press hard. Targets were set at 75% of maximum calculated from baseline assessment
	Counting to 15 with precise articulation five times (5 minutes)	Incorporate clear speech strategies from the first exercise into a semiautomatic speech task minimising the cognitive demands of the task and focusing on articulation
	Read 15 minimal pairs of words chosen based on sound errors (10 minutes)	Individualised articulation targets based on a phonetic analysis of sound error patterns and frequency of phoneme occurrence
Hierarchy		
Week 1	Read words and phrases (40 minutes)	Use clear speech while reading words and phrases to manage cognitive demands of the task and allow focus on articulation
Week 2	Read sentences and short answer conversation (40 minutes)	Use clear speech while reading sentences and short answer conversation to incorporate more precise articulation
Week 3	Structured dialogue and conversation (40 minutes)	Use clear speech during structured dialogue and short conversation to incorporate more precise articulation in functional communication
Week 4	Structured dialogue and conversation (40 minutes)	Use clear speech during structured dialogue and conversation
Cue	Say that as **clearly** as you can	Maintain the focus on precise articulation
Homework	A subset of daily exercises and assignments based on DS's activities (20 minutes)	Carryover and generalisation of treatment targets outside of the clinical environment

Iowa Oral Performance Instrument (IOPI) were obtained for the articulation treatment only. A paired-sample, one-tailed t-test was used to calculate statistical significance in the dependent variables post-treatment, and the effect size was used to determine clinical significance.

Therapeutic response to LSVT LOUD

DS made statistically and clinically significant increases in vocal intensity on all tasks except monologue following LSVT LOUD. It was challenging for DS to focus on speech targets during more cognitively demanding tasks such as picture description or monologue. DS's cognitive and linguistic deficits limited the length and complexity of the reading material used in treatment, and reading materials did not go beyond the single sentence level. It is also interesting to note that DS rarely initiated conversation exchanges at the onset of treatment. Therefore, treatment tasks were structured in a way to share the burden of communication to a greater extent with the clinician and increase initiation of conversation topics. DS was engaged throughout the treatment sessions, consistently completing homework and carryover tasks that were a critical part of the therapy. Table 4.3 shows mean vocal intensity (and standard deviation) measured at 40 cm and mean single-word intelligibility pre- and post-LSVT LOUD.

Therapeutic response to articulation therapy

Articulation treatment was undertaken because DS wanted to continue to work specifically on the clarity of her speech to improve articulation to be better understood in conversation. There was one month of withdrawal from treatment between LSVT LOUD and articulation therapy before voice and speech evaluations were re-administered. DS continued to be motivated and engaged throughout the treatment sessions, consistently completing homework and carryover tasks that were critical part of the therapy.

Table 4.3 Average and standard deviation pre- and post-LSVT LOUD for dB SPL and percent of single-word intelligibility

	Average Pre (SD)	Average Post (SD)	Pre-post mean difference	t-test	Effect size
Sustained vowel phonation dB SPL	81.83 (2.32)	87.13 (1.12)	5.30	0.03	0.82
Sentence reading dB SPL	65.77 (0.46)	70.20 (0.38)	4.43	0.00	0.98
Picture description dB SPL	66.70 (0.62)	69.10 (0.49)	2.40	0.02	0.90
Monologue dB SPL	65.87 (1.97)	69.60 (0.62)	3.73	0.07	0.79
Single-word intelligibility %	62.67 (4.16)	67.33 (5.03)	4.67	0.46	0.45

Table 4.4 Average and standard deviation pre- and post-articulation treatment for vocal dB SPL, IOPI kPa and percent of single-word intelligibility

	Average Pre (SD)	Average Post (SD)	Pre-post mean difference	t-test	Effect size
Sustained vowel phonation dB SPL	85.33 (2.09)	89.28 (0.62)	3.95	0.05	0.75
Sentence reading dB SPL	67.30 (1.42)	70.80 (0.80)	3.50	0.15	0.63
Picture description dB SPL	67.20 (1.21)	68.73 (1.09)	1.53	0.20	0.55
Monologue dB SPL	66.30 (2.04)	68.65 (0.62)	2.35	0.25	0.60
Lip pressure (kPa)	12.83 (1.50)	19.43 (1.26)	6.60	0.00	0.92
Tongue pressure (kPa)	21.75 (3.10)	49.00 (4.53)	27.30	0.00	0.96
Single-word intelligibility %	67.33 (1.15)	80.00 (2.00)	12.67	0.01	0.97

Results of the evaluations administered immediately before articulation therapy showed that DS had maintained vocal intensity gains achieved during LSVT LOUD, and she continued to make modest improvements in intensity during articulation therapy even though loudness was no longer the focus of treatment. Measurements of IOPI lip and tongue tip strength improved following treatment even though the goal of using the IOPI in therapy was to increase tactile and kinaesthetic awareness of the articulators as a reference for producing speech sounds clearly. There were also statistically and clinically significant improvements in single-word intelligibility following treatment that were greater than the gains following LSVT LOUD. Table 4.4 shows mean vocal intensity (and standard deviation) measured at 40 cm, mean kPa for lips and tongue and mean single-word intelligibility pre- and post-articulation treatment.

Discussion

Decreased intelligibility that results from dysarthria negatively impacts social participation and quality of life for people with DS. Dysarthria treatment could potentially improve communication and positively impact the ability of people with DS to benefit from cognitive-linguistic treatment and facilitate greater social participation and independence. This case report demonstrated that a young adult with DS made changes in her speech that had a positive impact on her communication.

She increased vocal intensity following LSVT LOUD, but there was not a significant increase in intelligibility, which had been one of her goals for treatment. Previous studies of LSVT LOUD treatment outcomes demonstrated a positive impact of treatment on articulation in addition to increased vocal intensity (Mahler & Ramig, 2012; Sapir et al., 2003). These studies reported outcomes of speech rehabilitation for adults with acquired dysarthria. Habilitation of speech for adults with DS who have a congenital dysarthria may not be as likely to achieve similar outcomes. There was a positive change in single-word intelligibility of 4.66% following LSVT LOUD, but it was not statistically or clinically significant and that is what motivated continuing treatment with a focus on articulation. DS demonstrated a 12.70% increase in single-word intelligibility following articulation treatment that was statistically significant (p = 0.01) and clinically significant (effect size = 0.86).

DS did better on highly structured speaking tasks, and it became clear early in treatment that she needed support to generalise treatment goals to conversation and carryover outside of the treatment room secondary to cognitive linguistic limitations. The structured dialogue activity was developed as a bridge from structured speech exercises to functional conversation that supported DS in conversation and social situations. Structured dialogues were based on DS's stated interests and goals for treatment, for example, going to a movie with friends, shopping for clothes, ordering a meal in a restaurant and job skills. Words and pictures were used in the dialogues along with printed words to facilitate DS's reading comprehension and maintain the flow of shared conversation exchanges. DS enjoyed structured dialogue activities because they facilitated more frequent initiation of conversation on her part. DS's parents stated in a post-treatment interview that DS's speech was louder after LSVT LOUD, clearer after articulation treatment and that she was using her strategies in social settings effectively. When asked to comment further, one parent reported, 'Treatment has helped her feel better about communication. Her confidence level has increased, and she is more comfortable engaging in conversation with others'.

Although people with DS share a common diagnosis, each person presents unique characteristics of communication. This case report showed that a young adult with DS who had dysarthria improved her communication even with the coexistence of cognitive-linguistic deficits. It also showed that improved communication led to greater social participation and confidence in communication skills. Future treatment studies should include following people for a longer period of time post-treatment to address ongoing communication needs.

Clinical message

It is not the purpose of this case report to suggest that all people with DS should receive dysarthria treatment nor is it to suggest a specific focus of treatment when dysarthria is addressed. A speech evaluation will identify the contribution of dysarthria to the communication challenges of a person with

DS, and clinician expertise will guide the selection of the most appropriate target of treatment if treatment of dysarthria is warranted. The results of this case report, as well as other studies, support the inclusion of principles of motor learning suggested by Maas et al. (2008) to obtain changes in speech behaviours that generalise outside of the treatment environment, whatever treatment focus is chosen.

Even though DS had dysarthria throughout her life, it had never been the focus of treatment prior to participation in this study. Instead, cognitive-linguistic skills had been targeted exclusively. The data from this case study suggest that speech-language pathologists should reappraise their approach to the treatment of motor speech disorders for this population given the longer life expectancy of people with DS today and the lack of services available for them as adults. The role of treating dysarthria in addition to cognitive-linguistic treatment as children and adults could be a tool for increasing success in verbal communication, facilitating cognitive-linguistic therapy and potentially increasing independence. Further treatment efficacy and effectiveness studies are needed to assess how children and adults with DS respond to specific motor speech treatments to meet ongoing communication needs.

Informed consent

This study was reviewed and approved by the Institutional Review Board at the University of Rhode Island. All information is deidentified for the purposes of this case report.

References

Carr, J. (2000). Intellectual and daily living skills of 30-year-olds with Down's syndrome: Continuation of a longitudinal study. *Journal of Applied Research and Intellectual Disability*, *13*, 1–16.

Carr, J., & Collins, S. (2018). 50 years with Down syndrome: A longitudinal study. *Journal of Applied Research and Intellectual Disability*, *31*, 743–750.

Docherty, J., & Reid, K. (2009). "What's the next stage?" Mothers of young adults with Down syndrome explore the path to independence: A qualitative investigation. *Journal of Applied Research in Intellectual Disabilities*, *22*, 458–467.

Down syndrome fact sheet: National Down Syndrome Society, www.ndss.org/about-down-syndrome/down-syndrome-facts/. (Retrieved 12–20–2020)

Dromey, C., Ramig, L.O., & Johnson, A. (1995). Phonatory and articulatory changes associated with increased vocal intensity in Parkinson disease: A case study. *Journal of Speech and Hearing Research*, *53*, 751–764.

Goldman, R., & Fristoe, M. (2000). Goldman-Fristoe test of articulation (2nd Ed.). Minneapolis, MN: NCS Pearson.

Jones, H.N., Crisp, K.D., Kuchibhatla, M., Mahler, L., Risoli, T., Jones, C., & Kishnani, P. (2019). Auditory-perceptual speech features in children with Down syndrome. *American Journal on Intellectual and Developmental Disabilities*, *124*(4), 324–338.

Kent, R.D., & Vorperian, H.K. (2013). Speech impairment in Down syndrome: A review. *Journal of Speech, Language, and Hearing Research, 56*(1), 178–210.

Kertesz, A. (2006). *Western aphasia battery-revised.* San Antonio, TX: Psychological Corporation.

Maas, E., Robin, D., Hula, S., Freedman, S., Wulf, G., Ballard, K., & Schmidt, R.A. (2008). Principles of motor learning in treatment of motor speech disorders. *American Journal of Speech-Language Pathology, 17,* 277–298.

Mahler, L., & Jones, H. (2012). Intensive treatment of dysarthria in two adults with Down syndrome. *Developmental Neurorehabilitation, 15,* 44–53.

Mahler, L., & Ramig, L.O. (2012). Intensive voice treatment of dysarthria secondary to stroke. *Journal of Clinical Linguistics and Phonetics, 26,* 681–694.

Mahler, L., Ramig, L.O., & Fox, C. (2015). Evidence-based treatment of voice and speech disorders in Parkinson disease. *Current Opinion in Otolaryngology & Head and Neck Surgery, 23,* 209–215.

O'Leary, D., Lee, A., O'Toole, C., & Gibbon, F. (2020). Perceptual and acoustic evaluation of speech production in Down syndrome: A case series. *Clinical Linguistics & Phonetics, 34,* 72–91.

Parker, S.E., Mai, C.T., Canfield, M.A., Rickard, R., Wang, Y., Meyer, R.E., . . . Correa, A. (2010). Updated national birth prevalence estimates for selected birth defects in the United States, 2004–2006. *Birth Defects Research: Part A: Clinical and Molecular Teratology, 88*(12), 1008–1016.

Ramig, L., Halpern, A., Spielman, J., Fox, C., & Freeman, K. (2018). Speech treatment in Parkinson's disease: Randomized control trial (RCT). *Movement Disorders, 33*(11), 1777–1791.

Randolph, C., Tierney, M.C., Mohr, E., & Chase, T.N. (1998). Repeatable battery for the assessment of neurological status (RBANS): Preliminary clinical validity. *Journal of Clinical Experimental Neuropsychology, 20*(3), 310–319. Doi: 10.1076/jcen.20.3.310.823

Sapir, S., Spielman, J., Ramig, L., Hinds, S., Countryman, S., Fox, C., & Story, B. (2003). Effects of intensive voice treatment (the Lee Silverman Voice Treatment [LSVT]) on ataxic dysarthria. *American Journal of Speech-Language Pathology, 12,* 387–399.

Sapir, S., Spielman, J.L., Ramig, L.O., Story, B.H., & Fox, C. (2007). Effects of intensive voice treatment (the Lee Silverman Voice Treatment), LSVT, on vowel articulation in dysarthric individuals with idiopathic Parkinson disease: Acoustic and perceptual findings. *Journal of Speech, Language, and Hearing Research, 50,* 899–912.

Smith, D.S. (2001). Health care management of adults with Down syndrome. *American Family Physician, 64(6),* 1031–1038.

Stoel-Gammon, C. (2001). Down syndrome phonology: Developmental patterns and intervention strategies. *Down Syndrome Research and Practice, 7,* 93–100.

Wild, A., Vorperian, H.K., Kent, R.D., Bolt, D.M., & Austin, D. (2018). Single-word speech intelligibility in children and adults with Down syndrome. *American Journal of Speech-Language Pathology, 27,* 222–236. Doi: 10.1044/2017_AJSLP-17-0002

Chapter 5

Be *Clear*, an intensive treatment for non-progressive dysarthria

A case report

Stacie Park, Deborah Theodoros, Emma Finch, and Elizabeth Cardell

Introduction

Traumatic brain injury (TBI) is a leading source of death and disability for individuals under the age of 40 years (Iaccarino et al. 2018). Of those who sustain a TBI, approximately 19–65% will present with dysarthria (Safaz et al. 2008; Yorkston et al. 1989). The complex nature of injury following TBI leads to a wide variation in the clinical presentation of speech disturbances, with all dysarthria subtypes possible (Duffy 2019). At present, the natural course and recovery of dysarthria following TBI is unclear (Morgan 2014). However, there is evidence to suggest that for many individuals who experience TBI, dysarthria is a chronic condition that may persist for many years post-initial injury (Zebenholzer & Oder 1998; Olver, Ponsford, & Curran 1996). As many individuals who experience TBI are young (Iaccarino et al. 2018), it is crucial that we develop optimal treatments to increase participation and minimise potential lifelong disability in this population.

Improved speech intelligibility remains a key treatment focus and goal for many individuals with TBI who present with dysarthria. Traditionally, the literature has advocated for individualising treatment for patients with dysarthria, with the speech-language pathologist (SLP) selecting specific treatment strategies depending on the nature and severity of each patient's speech disorder (Yorkston et al. 2010). Furthermore, contemporary practice guidelines in many countries call for individualised treatment to consider the impairment as well as activity and participation in line with The International Classification of Functioning, Disability and Health (ICF; WHO 2001). Traditional dysarthria treatment utilises a motor speech subsystem approach. Prior to commencing therapy, each component of the speech mechanism is individually assessed to determine which subsystems are not functioning optimally (Duffy 2019). Treatment strategies for therapy are then selected, accordingly. As individuals with dysarthria often present with deficits in multiple speech subsystems, treatment is usually multi-component. Therefore, a combination of treatment strategies, each of which may target a different speech subsystem, are generally practiced every session (Finch, Rumbach, & Park 2020;

DOI: 10.4324/9781003172536-5

Yorkston et al. 2010). Priority is given to those subsystems that will derive the greatest functional benefit or provide the greatest support for improvement in other aspects of speech (Duffy 2019).

Cognitive deficits are one of the most salient features of TBI, with studies consistently demonstrating that individuals with moderate-to-severe closed head injury perform significantly worse on neuropsychological testing relative to controls (Schretlen & Shapiro 2003; Fraser et al. 2019). As focal and diffuse damage resulting from TBI tends to concentrate in the anterior regions of the brain, including the frontal and temporal lobes (Bigler 2007; Scheid et al. 2003), deficits in attention, memory and executive function are frequently reported (Cristofori & Levin 2015). These cognitive deficits are often persistent, with individuals with TBI continuing to demonstrate poor performance on neuropsychological testing over 4.5 years post-injury (Ruttan et al. 2008).

Disturbances in cognitive functions can hinder an individual's ability to learn and maintain treatment strategies as well as diminish their capacity to self-monitor and modify their speech (Murdoch & Theodoros 2001). Therefore, treatment programmes focusing on implementing multiple treatment strategies may be difficult for individuals with TBI. Instead, targeting global behavioural changes that aim to enhance speech production in an integrated manner may be more appropriate. For example, adopting an external attentional focus on one aspect of speech (e.g. loudness) to achieve improved speech intelligibility may be a more suitable approach for people with non-progressive dysarthria following TBI.

'Clear speech' is one such strategy and refers to a speaking style where talkers spontaneously modify their habitual speech to enhance intelligibility for a listener. Typically, talkers employ clear speech when communicating in adverse conditions, such as when speaking in a noisy environment or speaking to somebody with a hearing loss. Studies in healthy talkers have found that speaking in an intentionally clear manner increases intelligibility by approximately 15–26 percentage points relative to habitual speech (Lam & Tjaden 2013). Preliminary stimulability trials in individuals with dysarthria secondary to TBI, idiopathic Parkinson's disease (PD) and multiple sclerosis (MS) have also shown that the use of clear speech can improve intelligibility in disordered speakers within a single assessment session (Beukelman et al. 2002; Tjaden, Sussman, & Wilding 2014).

Numerous studies have been conducted with healthy speakers to elucidate the acoustic-phonetic characteristics that contribute to the improved intelligibility associated with clear speech. These studies have identified numerous acoustic-phonetic markers of clear speech including decreased speech rate, prolonged phoneme durations, increased fundamental frequency and frequency range, increased pause frequency and duration, increased sound pressure level (SPL), increased vowel space area (VSA), increased consonant-to-vowel intensity ratios, decreased burst elimination and decreased alveolar flapping (Picheny, Durlach, & Braida 1986; Lam & Tjaden 2016). Initial investigations into the acoustic basis of clear speech in adults with PD and MS also have revealed that individuals with progressive dysarthria demonstrate many of the same speech production modifications as healthy speakers when cued to produce clear speech (Goberman & Elmer 2005; Lam & Tjaden 2016; Tjaden, Lam, & Wilding 2013). Based on these findings, it appears that clear speech may be a global variable that affects all speech subsystems, as well as the prosodic aspects of speech. As such, it may be a suitable compensatory technique for promoting speech intelligibility in individuals with dysarthria.

Based on the positive effects of clear speech on the speech intelligibility of healthy and disordered speakers, a new treatment programme for people with non-progressive dysarthria (*Be Clear*) was developed. The programme was designed to adhere to the principles of experience-dependent neuroplasticity (Kleim & Jones 2008) and motor learning (Maas et al. 2008), with treatment involving high-intensity practice of clear speech during salient connected speech tasks. A Phase I clinical trial examining the impact of *Be Clear* on the speech of eight individuals with dysarthria secondary to TBI and stroke reported positive results (Park et al. 2016). Following treatment, participants demonstrated significant short- and long-term improvements in word, sentence and conversational speech intelligibility. In addition, communication partner ratings of speech intelligibility and overall communicative function were significantly improved post-treatment. These results suggested that *Be Clear* may have potential as an effective intervention for non-progressive dysarthria. However, controlled studies are required to establish treatment efficacy.

The following case report is taken from the Park et al. (2016) study and demonstrates how, by adopting an external attentional focus on clear speech, individuals with TBI can achieve substantial changes across perceptual, acoustic, psychosocial well-being and everyday communication measures.

Case report: MP

MP was a 51-year-old male who had been working full-time as an audiovisual manager prior to his accident. He was married and had four young children. His interests included travel, cars, gardening, cooking and music.

Twelve months prior to referral, MP sustained a severe TBI in a motor vehicle accident. Early neuroimaging studies identified a displaced frontal skull fracture, extensive base of skull fracture, herniation of frontal lobe into left orbit, frontal contusions, left temporal extradural haematoma, right temporal lobe subdural haematoma and pneumocranium. Following 101 days of intensive and acute hospital management, MP was transferred to a neurorehabilitation ward where he remained for a further 159 days. Upon admission to the rehabilitation ward, MP completed an initial SLP assessment and was subsequently diagnosed with mild-to-moderate dysarthria characterised by poor respiratory support for speech, reduced pitch variability, harsh vocal quality and reduced articulatory precision. MP attended regular treatment sessions which focused on direct tasks such as respiratory support including diaphragmatic breathing, breath-voice coordination and sustained phonation; hierarchical speech drills; pitch glides with tactile feedback; lip and tongue drills to increase range of motion (ROM), coordination and speed; intonation and stress pattern drills and compensatory strategies related to self-monitoring and rating of speech. He also received regular SLP input for mild-to-moderate high-level cognitive communication for deficits across the areas of naming, verbal explanation, planning, auditory memory, auditory comprehension, reading, writing and numeracy. Upon discharge from the rehabilitation unit, MP was referred to the *Be Clear* research trial for ongoing management of his dysarthria.

Clinical findings

At the time of his referral to the *Be Clear* programme, MP was living at home with his family and was well supported by his wife. MP was ambulatory and mobilised using a four-wheel walker. He was receiving physiotherapy and occupational therapy and was enthusiastic about recommencing treatment to work on his speech deficits. Testing of cognitive function conducted 4.5 months prior to treatment identified deficits in orientation, memory and problem-solving.

An initial oro-motor examination (OME) revealed right-sided lower facial weakness, with reduced ROM during lip spreading, rounding and alternating movements. Lip seal was maintained for >15 seconds and was therefore judged by the assessing SLP to be adequate. MP's tongue was noted to deviate to the right at rest, with reduced ROM and coordination noted on protrusion/retraction, elevation/depression and lateralisation. Speed was moderately reduced during tongue lateralisation and alternating speech movements. Reduced articulatory precision was noted on lingual consonants during alternating movements. Laryngeal function was adversely affected, with harsh vocal quality and reduced loudness variability. Alternating motion rate (repeat/pa// pa/) and sequential motion rate (repeat/pataka/) were mildly reduced in speed.

Informal perceptual analysis of MP's conversational speech was characterised by decreased speech rate, imprecise consonant articulation, hypernasality, harsh voice, monopitch and monoloudness. These deviant perceptual speech features resulted in mild-to-moderate compromise in intelligibility during conversational speech. Based on the available medical information, perceptual judgement of speech samples and the OME, MP was diagnosed as having a mild-to-moderate spastic dysarthria.

Diagnostic assessment

To better understand the multidimensional nature of MP's speech impairment, assessments addressed the impairment, activity and participation domains of the ICF (WHO 2001). Assessments included perceptual measures of speech intelligibility, questionnaires pertaining to everyday communicative function and psychosocial well-being, perceptual ratings of deviant speech features and acoustic analysis.

Assessment of intelligibility using the Assessment of Intelligibility of Dysarthric Speech (AIDS) (Yorkston & Beukelman 1981) revealed 80.50% intelligibility for single words and 96.93% intelligibility at the sentence level. Reduced speech intelligibility was also reported in the home environment, with MP's wife indicating moderate difficulty in understanding his speech via a short informal communication partner questionnaire. The questionnaire revealed that MP's family frequently asked him to repeat himself and that they considered his overall speech function to be poor. Mild-to-moderate reductions in initiating conversations with familiar and unfamiliar communication partners were also noted. These changes to MP's speech appeared to have a negative impact on his psychosocial well-being as he scored 144 out of a possible 225 on the Dysarthria Impact Profile (DIP) (Walshe, Peach, & Miller 2009).

During the initial assessment, some additional speech samples were recorded. These included a reading of the Grandfather Passage (Darley, Aronson, & Brown 1975), reading of /b/ + vowel + /d/ (bVd) tokens centrally embedded in carrier sentences and a two-minute monologue. These samples were collected to monitor changes across a range of acoustic and perceptual outcome measures following intervention. Direct magnitude estimation (DME) was used to conduct auditory-perceptual analysis of MP's speech. Specifically, DME ratings of speech rate, articulatory precision and pitch variability were made from the Grandfather Passage samples. DME ratings of speech intelligibility were conducted on monologue speech samples. DME involves listeners making perceptual judgements in comparison to a 'standard' speech sample, which typically represents the approximate midpoint of a given perceptual continuum (Weismer & Laures 2002). Investigators assign the standard a value ('modulus'), typically 10 or 100. Listeners then judge the samples and assign them with a numerical value that is relative to the modulus. For example, when judging speech rate, a sample perceived to be twice as fast as the standard would be assigned a value of 200 whilst a sample perceived to be half the speed of the modulus would be assigned a value of 50 (Weismer & Laures 2002). Two experienced SLPs served as independent listeners for the DME scaling task.

Perceived changes in intelligibility during monologue were also provided by naive listeners using a paired comparisons rating task. Four listeners with no previous exposure to dysarthric speech were presented with pairs of speech samples in several different combinations including: (1) pre-treatment – post-treatment, (2) pre-treatment – follow-up (FU), (3) post-treatment – pre-treatment and (4) FU – pre-treatment. The listeners' task was to indicate whether the first or second sample of each pair was 'easier' to understand or whether there was no discernible difference. Listeners were blinded to the assessment interval (i.e. pre-treatment, post-treatment and FU).

Acoustic analysis was included in the *Be Clear* assessment protocol to provide an objective means of quantifying changes to the speech signal. MP's monologue and Grandfather Passage samples were used to examine changes in articulation rate (syllables/second), percent pause time, fundamental frequency and frequency range. To promote efficient batch processing of the speech samples, acoustic analysis was conducted using an automated PRAAT script (Vogel, Fletcher, & Maruff 2014). The bVd tokens produced by MP were used to investigate changes in VSA and vowel duration. This analysis was conducted manually using standard acoustic criteria.

All speech tasks were conducted twice during two separate assessment sessions, approximately two days apart, to account for effects from day-to-day variability in speech production. All assessment sessions were performed by a research SLP not directly involved in the delivery of the *Be Clear* treatment.

Therapeutic intervention

MP completed the standard *Be Clear* treatment protocol, as described in Park et al. (2016) (see Supplemental Material 5.1). All treatment sessions were delivered in an individual face-to-face format in a hospital outpatient setting. To ensure an understanding of the clear speech concept, MP completed an initial hour-long pre-practice session prior to moving into the intensive phase of the treatment protocol. During this session, MP watched video recordings of healthy non-dysarthric adults reading aloud a standard passage using both habitual and 'clear speech'. This was followed by a discussion regarding the differences between the two speaking modes that may have contributed to the observed improvements in speech clarity (e.g. exaggerated articulation). Next, MP read aloud the same standard passage while imitating the clear speech he had observed in the videos. The clinician provided specific knowledge of performance (KP) feedback on MP's speech production during this session to shape clearer speech and determine the most effective speaking strategy to produce more intelligible speech.

A variety of cues have been used in the literature to elicit clear speech. For example, 'speak clearly', 'hyperarticulate' and 'speak to someone with a hearing impairment' (Lam, Tjaden, & Wilding 2012). Through stimulability testing, it was determined that MP's most effective 'clear speech' strategy was to use exaggerated articulation.

Following this pre-practice session, MP commenced the intensive phase of the *Be Clear* programme, completing four one-hour treatment sessions per week for four weeks. Each session followed a standard format which included:

(1) a brief pre-practice session to shape MP's speech production and elicit a small number of correct productions prior to moving into the practice phase of the session;

(2) block practice of 20 functional phrases covering biographical information, service requests and high-frequency everyday phrases (five repetitions); and
(3) random practice of picture description, reading and conversational speech tasks.

During the second half of the treatment session, MP was allowed three attempts to achieve clear speech for a given stimulus item before moving onto the next randomly selected task. See supplementary resources for further information regarding the structure of individual treatment sessions.

During the 'practice' phase of each session, the treating clinician provided MP with knowledge of results (KR) feedback as to whether his speech output was considered clear or unclear. Providing KR feedback during treatment may enhance the retention of trained speech skills and further promote the adoption of an external attentional focus on clear speech (Ballard et al. 2012). To assist MP in developing his ability to self-monitor the clarity of his speech signal, his speech was audio recorded during the session and played back intermittently. MP then rated his speech clarity on a scale of 1 (unclear: speech completely unintelligible) to 10 (clear: all sounds articulated clearly).

To ensure treatment was salient, all treatment stimuli were personalised and created by the treating clinician based on MP's unique interests and functional needs. To further increase treatment intensity, MP was required to complete independent daily homework involving practice of his functional phrases, reading aloud, picture description and conversation. MP was encouraged to audio record his speech during these tasks to self-monitor speech clarity and modify where necessary. In addition, MP completed daily carry-over tasks designed to promote the transfer of his clear speech to everyday situations (e.g. talking on the phone, ordering a coffee at a cafe and requesting information about items in a shop). Compliance with home practice was monitored during each treatment session via verbal check-in. Treatment stimuli were presented on a computer screen via a PowerPoint presentation. Similarly, homework was saved as a PowerPoint presentation and provided to MP on a USB stick. Presenting treatment stimuli in this manner increased the ease of presenting treatment materials in a random order.

Following the completion of the four-week *Be Clear* programme, MP was required to continue to practice therapy activities at home for ten minutes a day, three to five days until the follow-up assessment sessions were conducted.

Follow-up and outcomes

To evaluate treatment outcomes, all perceptual, acoustic and everyday communication assessments were conducted twice immediately post-treatment and at three months post-treatment (FU).

MP was highly motivated to work on his speech deficits and participated enthusiastically during all treatment sessions. He attended all 16 treatment sessions as scheduled and reported high compliance with home practice. MP appeared to tolerate the *Be Clear* treatment schedule well and never expressed any concerns that structure of the programme was too intense.

The treating clinician noted that prompts to speak clearly resulted in marked articulatory exaggeration, leading to perceptual improvements in articulatory precision and a decrease in speech rate. Following the completion of the *Be Clear* programme, MP demonstrated marked improvements in speech intelligibility on both formal and informal measures. These improvements were associated with acoustic changes including decreased articulatory rate, increased vowel duration, increased percent pause time and increased VSA. However, changes in these acoustic parameters were not reflected in DME ratings. MP demonstrated improved psychosocial well-being post-treatment, as measured on the DIP. MP reported improvements in his ability to communicate with his family upon completion of the *Be Clear* programme, about which he was very satisfied.

Perceptual results

MP demonstrated improved speech intelligibility according to listeners on different speech tasks. With respect to the AIDS, there are currently no published data available to indicate what may be considered a minimal, clinically important change in word or sentence intelligibility on this outcome measure. Therefore, for the purposes of the present case, the criterion for clinically significant change was set with respect to the test–retest speaker variability reported in the AIDS manual (Yorkston & Beukelman 1981). As such, the criterion for clinically significant change was set at ±3.2% for word intelligibility and ±8.6% for sentence intelligibility. Based on these figures, MP demonstrated a clinically significant improvement of 6.08% in word intelligibility immediately post-treatment. MP's word level intelligibility increased further at FU, improving by 18% to give a word intelligibility score of 98.5%. Despite these word level intelligibility gains, MP did not show clinically significant changes in sentence intelligibility. This is likely due to ceiling effects, with MP 96.93% intelligible at sentence level prior to treatment. It has been suggested that ongoing recovery for individuals with mild dysarthria may not be signalled by further improvements in intelligibility on this assessment (Yorkston & Beukelman 1981).

The improvements on the AIDS were supported by improvements on informal measures of speech intelligibility, including the paired comparisons rating task. The four naïve listeners unanimously rated MP's speech as being more intelligible immediately post-treatment when compared to pre-treatment speech samples. Furthermore, all listeners indicated this improvement was maintained at follow-up. Given that listeners on this rating task had no prior exposure to dysarthric speech, it is anticipated that members of the community would also perceive improvements in MP's intelligibility post-treatment.

Meaningful improvements in speech intelligibility, as perceived by trained listeners, also were reported on the DME rating task immediately post-treatment and at FU. Whilst MP demonstrated a trend towards decreased speech rate and increased pitch variability on DME ratings, these changes were less than 1 standard deviation from the pre-treatment mean and were therefore not deemed meaningful (Sapir et al. 2003).

Acoustic results

The trends noted on perceptual ratings of MP's speech were corroborated by acoustic outcome measures. For instance, the perceived decrease in speech rate recorded during the DME ratings was represented acoustically by a meaningful decrease in articulatory rate, increase in vowel duration and an increase in percent pause immediately post-treatment. Changes in articulatory rate were maintained at FU. The perceived perceptual improvements in pitch variability were also associated with increased pitch range on acoustic outcome measures immediately post-treatment and at FU.

Despite not demonstrating meaningful changes in articulatory precision on the DME rating task, MP increased his VSA immediately post-treatment. However, this change was not maintained at follow-up. An increase in VSA may be indicative of increased articulatory displacement (Mefferd 2015) and thus improved articulatory precision. There is preliminary evidence to suggest that these changes in VSA may be associated with improved speech intelligibility in dysarthric speakers (Hustad & Lee 2008; Liu, Tsao, & Kuhl 2005). Therefore, such changes may have further contributed to MP's improved ratings of speech intelligibility on formal and informal outcome measures. Taken together, the results of the acoustic analysis revealed that MP demonstrated a number of temporal, prosodic and articulatory changes that are consistent with clear speech production in healthy speakers (Lam, Tjaden, & Wilding 2012; Picheny, Durlach, & Braida 1986; Whitfield & Goberman 2017).

Psychosocial well-being and everyday communication outcomes

Improvements in speech intelligibility were accompanied by improvements in psychosocial well-being, with MP's total impact score on the DIP improving by 33 points immediately post-treatment and 31 points at FU. MP's primary communication partner also reported improvements in four of the five parameters investigated on the everyday communication questionnaire including an improved ability to understand the speaker, a decrease in the number of repetitions requested, improved initiation of conversation with familiar speakers and improved overall speech quality. In fact, MP's wife reported that his intelligibility had improved to the extent that immediate family members no longer had to ask him to repeat himself. MP also reported being very pleased with his improved ability to communicate with his family, stating that before the treatment he had often felt very frustrated by his wife and children 'nagging' him to repeat himself.

Overall, MP reported that he enjoyed participating in the *Be Clear* programme and that he was pleased with the improvements in his speech. The improvements in intelligibility reported by his family may be indicative of improved participation in the home environment and suggest that MP was successful in generalising his clear speech to communicative contexts outside clinical or practise settings. Improvements in intelligibility were associated with improvements in psychosocial well-being post-treatment. This result is promising given the need for SLPs to treat their clients in a holistic manner that extends beyond the underlying neuromotor deficit to address the social and psychological consequences of their condition (Ross, Bickford, & Scholten 2018).

Discussion

This case report details the effects of *Be Clear* on the speech of MP, a middle-aged man presenting with non-progressive dysarthria secondary to severe TBI. Following treatment, MP demonstrated both short- and long-term improvements across a range of perceptual, acoustic, psychosocial and everyday communication outcome measures. The results of this case are consistent with previous findings that clear speech can enhance speech intelligibility in adults with non-progressive dysarthria (Beukelman et al. 2002). As such, this case report lends further support for the use of clear speech as a treatment technique for improving speech production in adults with dysarthria due to TBI.

Participant eligibility for Be Clear

The present case study is concerned with the remediation of speech deficits following severe TBI. However, preliminary evidence suggests that the use of clear speech may also improve intelligibility in individuals experiencing dysarthria secondary to stroke, PD and MS (Beukelman et al. 2002; Park et al. 2016; Tjaden, Sussman, & Wilding 2014). As such, the *Be Clear* programme may prove beneficial for patient populations beyond those discussed in the present case. To ascertain an individual's suitability for the *Be Clear* programme, it is recommended that clinicians establish participant stimulability for clear speech before trialling the programme on an individual basis. Stimulability testing should be conducted across a range of speech tasks to determine whether the individual is likely to benefit from clear speech and establish their capacity to hear differences in speech output. If, by the end of this testing, the individual with dysarthria has failed to demonstrate any clear speech benefit, then the *Be Clear* programme should be discontinued and an alternate treatment should be pursued. Potential participants must also have enough physical reserve to tolerate the intensive nature of the *Be Clear* treatment protocol. Individuals who are in the early stages of recovery following acquired brain injury and are still experiencing high levels of fatigue may need to postpone commencing *Be Clear* until their stamina improves.

Preliminary perceptual and acoustic analyses indicate that the *Be Clear* programme may be beneficial for individuals who can achieve improved speech intelligibility by adopting a single strategy such as exaggerated articulation. However, alternate treatment techniques should be considered for individuals whose primary impairment occur in specific subsystems of the speech mechanism. For example, individuals with significant respiratory-phonatory or velopharyngeal dysfunction may need to complete intensive impairment-based treatment to address these deficits prior to completing the *Be Clear* programme. Furthermore, some individuals who complete the *Be Clear* programme may require additional treatment to target speech features for which the programme appeared to have limited effect (e.g. naturalness).

Delivery of the **Be Clear** *programme*

The *Be Clear* programme differs from many published dysarthria treatment techniques due to its strong theoretical grounding in the principles of neuroplasticity and motor learning. This is exemplified by the programme's intensive and repetitive treatment schedule, exclusive use of complex and salient connected speech tasks, external attentional focus on the speech signal, use of random practice and provision of KR feedback (Park et al. 2016). Research in both animal and human models has shown that applying these principles to behavioural treatment techniques may improve the retention and transfer of trained skills (Bislick et al. 2012; Kleim & Jones 2008). As such, the unique format of the *Be Clear* programme may have contributed to MP's success post-treatment.

Research into the effects of the *Be Clear* programme adds to a growing body of evidence indicating that meaningful improvements in speech production may be best achieved through the use of intensive treatment protocols (Levy et al. 2020; Wenke, Theodoros, & Cornwell 2011). As such, modifications to the intensity of the *Be Clear* programme is strongly discouraged. To facilitate high-intensity dysarthria treatment in the busy clinical setting, SLPs may need to consider sharing the management of individual clients between clinician caseloads or across SLP services (e.g. shared delivery of *Be Clear* between hospital outpatient and community services). The prescriptive nature of the programme also means that it may be suitable for use in student led clinics under the supervision of an SLP trained in this approach.

Assessment of treatment outcomes

Outcome measures for evaluating the effectiveness of *Be Clear* should reflect the programmes' goal of improving speech intelligibility through global behavioural changes in speech production. As such, any proposed assessment battery should include a formal measure of speech intelligibility (e.g. AIDS and Sentence Intelligibility Test (Yorkston, Beukelman, & Tice 1996)), conversational speech recording for perceptual analysis of clarity and a measure of functional communication (e.g. Communication Effectiveness Index-Modified (Donovan et al. 2008)). It is preferable to have an unfamiliar listener (e.g. non-treating clinician or therapy assistant) conduct perceptual ratings of speech intelligibility and clarity as the treating SLP's judgements may become biased by familiarity with the client's speech over the course of treatment. In addition, questionnaires such as DIP can be easily completed in the client's own time and add valuable information pertaining to the psychosocial impact of dysarthria on the individual. All outcome measures should be complete at least once pre- and post-treatment.

Conclusion

Overall, it appears that the *Be Clear* programme may be a useful technique for addressing the activity limitations experienced by individuals with non-progressive dysarthria by improving speech intelligibility. However, the following key points should be considered before commencing treatment:

* Client stimulability for clear speech should be established prior to completing the *Be Clear* programme. Client's must also possess adequate physical reserve and cognitive capacity to complete the programme.
* The *Be Clear* programmes intensive treatment schedule should be maintained. This may involve trialling shared care arrangements between clinicians or SLP services to facilitate the delivery of the programme in the busy clinical context.
* All outcome measures must be completed at least once pre- and post-treatment and should examine the individual's everyday communication skills.

References

Ballard, KJ, Smith, HD, Paramatmuni, D, McCabe, P, Theodoros, DG, & Murdoch, BE 2012, 'Amount of kinematic feedback affects learning of speech motor skills', *Motor Control*, vol. 16, no. 1, pp. 106–119.

Beukelman, DR, Fager, S, Ullman, C, Hanson, E, & Logemann, J 2002, 'The impact of speech supplementation and clear speech on the intelligibility and speaking rate of people with traumatic brain injury', *Journal of Medical Speech-Language Pathology*, vol. 10, no. 4, pp. 237–242.

Bigler, ED 2007, 'Anterior and middle cranial fossa in traumatic brain injury: Relevant neuroanatomy and neuropathology in the study of neuropsychological outcome', *Neuropsychology*, vol. 21, no. 5, pp. 515–531.

Bislick, LP, Weir, PC, Spencer, K, Kendall, D, & Yorkston, KM 2012, 'Do principles of motor learning enhance retention and transfer of speech skills? A systematic review', *Aphasiology*, vol. 26, no. 5, pp. 709–728.

Cristofori, I & Levin, HS 2015, 'Traumatic brain injury and cognition', *Handbook of Clinical Neurology*, vol. 128, pp. 579–611.

Darley, FL, Aronson, AE, & Brown, JR 1975, *Motor speech disorders*, Saunders, Philadelphia.

Donovan, NJ., Kendall, DL, Young, ME, & Rosenbek, JC 2008, 'The communicative effectiveness survey: Preliminary evidence of construct validity', *American Journal of Speech-Language Pathology*, vol. 17, no. 4, pp. 335–347.

Duffy, JR 2019, *Motor speech disorders: Substrates, differential diagnosis, and management*, 4th edn, Elsevier, St Louis.

Finch, E, Rumbach, AF, & Park, S 2020. 'Speech pathology management of non-progressive dysarthria: A systematic review of the literature', *Disability and Rehabilitation*, vol. 42, no. 3, pp. 296–306.

Fraser, EE, Downing, MG, Biernacki, K, McKenzie, DP, & Ponsford, JL 2019, 'Cognitive reserve and age predict cognitive recovery after mild to severe traumatic brain injury', *Journal of Neurotrauma*, vol. 36, no. 19, pp. 2753–2761.

Goberman, AM, & Elmer, LW 2005, 'Acoustic analysis of clear versus conversational speech in individuals with Parkinson disease', *Journal of Communication Disorders*, vol. 38, no. 3, pp. 215–230.

Hustad, KC, & Lee, J 2008, 'Changes in speech production associated with alphabet supplementation', *Journal of Speech, Language, and Hearing Research*, vol. 51, no. 6, pp. 1438–1450.

Iaccarino, C, Carretta, A, Nicolosi, F, & Morselli, C 2018, 'Epidemiology of severe traumatic brain injury', *Journal of Neurosurgical Sciences*, vol. 62, no. 5, pp. 535–541.

Kleim, JA, & Jones, TA 2008, 'Principles of experience-dependent neural plasticity: Implications for rehabilitation after brain damage', *Journal of Speech, Language, and Hearing Research*, vol. 51, no. 1, pp. S225–S239.

Lam, J, & Tjaden, K 2013, 'Intelligibility of clear speech: Effect of instruction', *Journal of Speech, Language, and Hearing Research*, vol. 56, no. 5, pp. 1429–1440.

Lam, J, & Tjaden, K 2016, 'Clear speech variants: An acoustic study in Parkinson's disease', *Journal of Speech, Language, and Hearing Research*, vol. 59, pp. 631–646.

Lam, J, Tjaden, K, & Wilding, G 2012, 'Acoustics of clear speech: Effect of instruction', *Journal of Speech, Language, and Hearing Research*, vol. 55, no. 6, pp. 1807–1821.

Levy ES, Moya-Gale G, Chang YM, Freeman K, Forrest K, Brin M, & Ramig L 2020, 'The effects of intensive speech treatment on intelligibility in Parkinson's disease: A randomised controlled trial', *EClinicalMedicine*, vol. 24, pp. 100429.

Liu, H-M, Tsao, F-M, & Kuhl, PK 2005, 'The effect of reduced vowel working space on speech intelligibility in Mandarin-speaking young adults with cerebral palsy', *The Journal of the Acoustical Society of America*, vol. 117, no. 6, pp. 3879–3889.

Maas, E, Robin, DA, Austermann Hula, SN, Freedman, SE, Wulf, G, Ballard, KJ, & Schmidt, RA 2008, 'Principles of motor learning in treatment of motor speech disorders', *American Journal of Speech-Language Pathology*, vol. 17, no. 3, pp. 277–298.

Mefferd, A 2015, 'Articulatory-to-acoustic relations in talkers with dysarthria: A first analysis', *Journal of Speech, Language, and Hearing Research*, vol. 58, no. 3, pp. 576–589.

Morgan, A 2014, 'Dysarthria in children and adults with traumatic brain injury', in S McDonald, L Togher, & C Code (Eds.), 2nd edn, *Social and communication disorders following traumatic brain injury*, Psychology Press, London.

Murdoch, BE, & Theodoros, DG 2001, *Traumatic brain injury: Associated speech, language, and swallowing disorders*, Singular Publishing Group, San Diego, CA.

Olver, JH, Ponsford, J, & Curran, C 1996, 'Outcome following traumatic brain injury: A comparison between 2 and 5 years after injury', *Brain Injury*, vol. 10, no. 11, pp. 841–848.

Park, S, Theodoros, D, Finch, E, & Cardell, E 2016, 'Be clear: A new intensive speech treatment for adults with nonprogressive dysarthria', *American Journal of Speech-Language Pathology*, vol. 25, no. 1, pp. 97–110.

Picheny, MA, Durlach, NI, & Braida, LD 1986, 'Speaking clearly for the hard of hearing: II: Acoustic characteristics of clear and conversational speech', *Journal of Speech and Hearing Research*, vol. 29, no. 4, pp. 434–446.

Ross, K, Bickford, J, & Scholten, I 2018, 'The ICF as a "way of thinking": An exploratory study of Australian speech-language pathologists' perceptions regarding application of the International Classification of Functioning, Disability and Health', *Journal of Clinical Practice in Speech-Language Pathology*, vol. 20, no. 3, pp. 111–120.

Ruttan, L, Martin, K, Liu, A, Colella, B, & Green, RE 2008, 'Long-term cognitive outcome in moderate to severe traumatic brain injury: A meta-analysis examining timed and untimed tests at 1 and 4.5 or more years after injury', *Archives of Physical Medicine and Rehabilitation*, vol. 89, no. 12, pp. S69–S76.

Safaz, I, Alaca, R, Yasar, E, Tok, F, & Yilmaz, B 2008, 'Medical complications, physical function and communication skills in patients with traumatic brain injury: A single centre 5-year experience', *Brain Injury*, vol. 22, no. 10, pp. 733–739.

Sapir, S, Spielman, J, Ramig, LO, Hinds, SL, Countryman, S, Fox, C, & Story, B 2003, 'Effects of intensive voice treatment (the Lee Silverman Voice Treatment [LSVT]) on ataxic dysarthria: A case study', *American Journal of Speech-Language Pathology*, vol. 12, pp. 387–399.

Scheid, R, Preul, C, Gruber, O, Wiggins, C, & Von Cramon, DY 2003, 'Diffuse axonal injury associated with chronic traumatic brain injury: Evidence from T2*-weighted gradient-echo imaging at 3 T', *American Journal of Neuroradiology*, vol. 24, no. 6, pp. 1049–1056.

Schretlen, DJ, & Shapiro, AM 2003, 'A quantitative review of the effects of traumatic brain injury on cognitive functioning', *International Review of Psychiatry*, vol. 15, no. 4, pp. 341–349.

Tjaden, K, Lam, J, & Wilding, G 2013, 'Vowel acoustics in Parkinson's disease and multiple sclerosis: Comparison of clear, loud, and slow speaking conditions', *Journal of Speech, Language, and Hearing Research*, vol. 56, no. 5, pp. 1485–1502.

Tjaden, K, Sussman, JE, & Wilding, GE 2014, 'Impact of clear, loud, and slow speech on scaled intelligibility and speech severity in Parkinson's disease and multiple sclerosis', *Journal of Speech, Language, and Hearing Research*, vol. 57, pp. 779–792.

Vogel, AP, Fletcher, J, & Maruff, P 2014, 'The impact of task automaticity on speech in noise', *Speech Communication*, vol. 65, pp. 1–8.

Walshe, M, Peach, RK, & Miller, N 2009, 'Dysarthria impact profile: Development of a scale to measure psychosocial effects', *International Journal of Language & Communication Disorders*, vol. 44, no. 5, pp. 693–715.

Weismer, G, & Laures, JS 2002, 'Direct magnitude estimates of speech intelligibility in dysarthria: Effects of a chosen standard', *Journal of Speech, Language, and Hearing Research*, vol. 45, no. 3, pp. 421–433.

Wenke, RJ, Theodoros, DG, & Cornwell, P 2011, 'A comparison of the effects of the Lee Silverman Voice Treatment and traditional therapy on intelligibility, perceptual speech features, and everyday communication in nonprogressive dysarthria', *Journal of Medical Speech-Language Pathology*, vol. 19, no. 4, pp. 1–24.

Whitfield, JA, & Goberman, AM 2017, 'Articulatory-acoustic vowel space: Associations between acoustic and perceptual measures of clear speech', *International Journal of Speech-Language Pathology*, vol. 19, no. 2, pp. 184–194.

World Health Organization 2001, *ICF, international classification of functioning, disability and health*, Short version, Geneva: World Health Organization.

Yorkston, KM, & Beukelman, DR 1981, *Assessment of intelligibility of dysarthric speech*, Pro-Ed, Austin, Tex.

Yorkston, KM, Beukelman, DR, Strand, EA, & Hakel, M 2010, *Management of motor speech disorders in children and adults*, 3rd edn, Pro-Ed, Austin, Tex.

Yorkston, K, Beukelman, DR, & Tice, R 1996, *Sentence intelligibility test*, Tice Technologies, Lincoln, NE.

Yorkston, KM, Honsinger, MJ, Mitsuda, PM, & Hammen, V 1989, 'The relationship between speech and swallowing disorders in head-injured patients', *The Journal of Head Trauma Rehabilitation*, vol. 4, no. 4, pp. 1–16.

Zebenholzer, K, & Oder, W 1998, 'Neurological and psychosocial sequelae 4 and 8 years after severe craniocerebral injury: A catamnestic study', *Wiener Klinische Wochenschrift*, vol. 110, no. 7, pp. 253–261.

Chapter 6

Be *Clear online* – a telepractice application for dysarthria rehabilitation

Brooke-Mai Whelan, Rachael Rietdijk, Deborah Theodoros, and Annie J Hill

Introduction

Telepractice is the application of information and telecommunications technology to deliver clinical services over a distance by linking client, caregiver or any person(s) responsible for delivering care to the client to a clinician, for the purpose of assessment, intervention, consultation and/or supervision (Speech Pathology Australia 2014). Whilst telepractice is the preferred term used by Speech Pathology Australia, other terms such as telehealth, teletherapy, telerehabilitation and teleSpeech may be used. Telepractice is a closed loop, which requires a connection between the client, caregiver or other person delivering care to the client and the clinician. Therefore, telepractice does not include independently accessed health apps. Telepractice forms part of a larger concept known as e-Health, which is a term given to electronic processes and communication technology that supports healthcare practice, for example, an electronic health record system.

The use of telepractice in dysarthria intervention has a history of over 20 years since first described by Duffy, Werven & Aronson (1997). Dysarthria is a chronic condition requiring long-term speech-language pathology (SLP) management. Interventions for dysarthria commonly involve frequent sessions, combined with independent at-home practice. Given these factors, telepractice may offer advantages over in-person services.

The feasibility of using telepractice to deliver high-intensity practice in dysarthria interventions has been demonstrated for the Lee Silverman Voice Treatment (LSVT LOUD) (Ramig et al. 2001), which requires four sessions per week (Covert, Slevin & Hatterman 2018; Theodoros, Hill & Russell 2016). High-intensity intervention can also be supported using asynchronous telepractice models, in which clients engage in frequent independent practice, which is monitored by the speech-language pathologist (SLP). For example, a dysarthria treatment programme involving four sessions of independent practice per week, which is reviewed and adjusted asynchronously by a clinician, has been successfully trialled (Beijer et al. 2010a).

DOI: 10.4324/9781003172536-6

Telepractice can address issues of continuity of care over the long term in the management of dysarthria, when there may be barriers to in-person attendance, such as transport issues, fatigue or geographical distance. Furthermore, management may be enhanced by using telepractice to provide intervention directly into the home or work environments, which are more ecologically valid than a clinical setting. Research has found that clients in a telepractice model of dysarthria intervention had significantly fewer missed appointments than those receiving in-person intervention (Covert, Slevin & Hatterman 2018), which may translate to clients receiving a full dose of intervention, thus potentially enhancing treatment effectiveness. Telepractice can also be used to support the sustainability of treatment outcomes over the long term and has successfully been used in group maintenance programmes (Quinn et al. 2019). Further benefits for patients receiving dysarthria therapy via telepractice include reduced costs associated with lost income and transport (Saiyed et al. 2020), the convenience of eliminating the need for travel (Griffin et al. 2018) and equitable access to services for people in regional and rural areas (Theodoros, Hill & Russell 2016). Research has found high levels of client satisfaction with telepractice interventions, even for clients who are initially uncertain about engaging with this mode of service delivery (Chan et al. 2019).

Recently, there has been an increase in adoption of telepractice for SLP services internationally in response to restrictions related to the COVID-19 pandemic (Feeney et al. 2021). Although this rapid transition was challenging for SLPs (Fong, Tsai & Yiu 2021), the use of telepractice in managing dysarthria is well supported by research. Non-inferiority assessment and treatment trials have shown comparability between telepractice and in-person dysarthria management via videoconferencing (Constantinescu et al. 2010; Griffin et al. 2018; Hill et al. 2006; Hill et al. 2009; Theodoros et al. 2003). The use of telepractice in dysarthria management has been validated across different approaches to assessment and management, including the Assessment of Intelligibility of Dysarthric Speech (AIDS) (Yorkston & Beukelman 1984) validated by Hill et al. (2006, 2009) and Constantinescu et al. (2010), Frenchay Dysarthria Assessment (Enderby 1983) validated by Hill et al. (2006) and Theodoros et al. (2003), perceptual speech ratings (Hill et al. 2006), LSVT LOUD (Theodoros, Hill & Russell 2016) and pitch limiting voice treatment (Beijer et al. 2010a).

The model of telepractice most commonly described in these studies is real-time videoconferencing between the clinician and the client, using customised telerehabilitation systems, such as eHab 2.0 (Theodoros, Hill & Russell 2016), or specialised videoconferencing equipment (Covert, Slevin & Hatterman 2018). Generic videoconferencing platforms such as Adobe Connect (Dias et al. 2016), WhatsApp (Chan et al. 2019), Facetime (Griffin et al. 2018) and Skype (Howell, Tripoliti & Pring 2009) have also been used for telepractice. Some studies also use store-and-forward capabilities to record and transmit high-quality speech samples to the clinician (Constantinescu et al. 2011;

Theodoros, Hill & Russell 2016). Most studies have involved individual telepractice sessions between a clinician and client; however, group sessions are also feasible (Quinn et al. 2019). Asynchronous telepractice is a different model involving clinicians monitoring a client's self-managed therapeutic programme, with minimal real-time contact (Beijer et al. 2010b).

This chapter will outline clinical considerations related to using telepractice for dysarthria management and illustrate the process of adapting intervention for online delivery using the example of the programme, *Be Clear*. This programme is described separately in Chapter 5 in this text.

Clinical considerations in delivering dysarthria management via telepractice

To ensure successful and effective implementation of telepractice in dysarthria management, careful planning and preparation is required by the clinician. Clinical considerations include:

1   Examination of the evidence base for the delivery of the intervention via telepractice. Has the intervention been trialled for delivery via telepractice? If an evidence base exists, are there specific requirements for achieving equivalency with in-person delivery? Examples might include specific features in the technology platform such as screen sharing or audio capture with store-and-forward capabilities.

2   Client attributes: It is important to consider the client's suitability for telepractice, including their physical and sensory capabilities, any requirements for appropriate cultural and linguistic support, and attention and motivation levels.

3   Location: Where will the intervention be delivered from (service provider location) and to (client location)? In identifying suitable locations, factors such as privacy, adequate lighting and quietness should be considered. Suitable locations may include the client's home, a community facility such as a private room in a library or health facility.

4   Training requirements: Training is essential for both clinicians and clients. Clinicians should ensure that they are familiar with all functions of the technology, be competent in its use through practice with a peer and be able to perform basic troubleshooting prior to delivery of a service. Clients (and their support person if necessary) require step-by-step instructions in written format to operate and troubleshoot the technology and the opportunity to engage in a practice session with the clinician.

5   Support: Considerations span both personal support for the intervention itself in the form of a support person at the client end and technology support depending upon the client's skills and needs. The client's access to technology and internet connectivity should be assessed and ideally

a trial conducted before intervention commences. Ongoing technology support should be available for both clients and clinicians. As part of the consent process, the client should be made aware of any deviation from mandatory privacy or security regulations.

6   Technology selection: It is essential that the technology used in dysarthria management is fit for purpose. This requires a systematic and comprehensive task analysis that moves from the clinical need and interaction through to interrogation of the technical features required to enable that clinical interaction. The steps involved in a task analysis include:

   a   Details of the clinical tasks that will occur within a typical session (e.g. reading aloud a functional phrase with feedback to the client on their intelligibility)
   b   Stimuli required to be presented to the client (e.g. display of functional phrases on client monitor)
   c   Client response (e.g. client reads aloud the functional phrase)
   d   Capture of client response (audio capture of client attempt)
   e   Clinician response to client action (feedback to client, e.g. verbal feedback and playback of client's audio file)
   f   Technical features required to enable the clinical interaction (e.g. videoconferencing for real-time interaction between client and clinician, display of functional phrases via screen share or remote control of client's computer, capture of client's verbal response and store-and-forward to clinician).
   g   Evaluate the technology options against the task analysis requirements. Ideally, a simulation trial would enable the clinician to evaluate whether the technology platforms have the required technical features (e.g. ability to screen share, and draw or annotate on a whiteboard capability to capture high-quality audio at client end (for intelligibility or acoustic analyses) and forward to clinician.

7   Digital resources: The resources needed for the intervention (e.g. functional phrases, images for picture description) should be developed and digitally stored for ready access during the telepractice sessions.

8   Evaluation of telepractice delivery of intervention: Depending upon the needs of the client, clinician and overall service, a range of outcome measures should be used to comprehensively evaluate the use of telepractice to deliver the intervention. Outcomes measured may include clinical and quality of life outcomes, client and clinician satisfaction, service metrics (e.g. time spent in consultation and intensity of intervention received) and costs from the perspective of both service provider and client.

Delivery of Be Clear *dysarthria intervention* *via telepractice*

TM, the focus of this chapter, participated in a larger research project evaluating the feasibility and acceptability of an online adaptation of the *Be Clear* programme developed by Park et al. (2016). The vignette describes how the *Be Clear* speech treatment programme was successfully adapted and delivered online.

Case report

TM was a 45-year-old male motor mechanic who sustained a traumatic brain injury following strangulation injury resulting in bilateral cerebellar infarcts. Resultant sequelae included: severe dysphagia (requiring enteral feeding), mild-to-moderate cognitive-communication impairment, severe dysarthria, balance impairment and motor incoordination. TM received acute medical care in a metropolitan hospital for 65 days, following which he was transferred to a brain injury rehabilitation unit for 221 days. On discharge home, he was referred to a transitional rehabilitation service. A nine-week block of SLP intervention was provided from this service, which focused upon Continuous Positive Airway Pressure (CPAP) treatment for the remediation of moderate-to-severe hypernasality and improving intelligibility with unfamiliar communication partners using clear speech strategies (i.e. rate reduction and over-articulation).

Twelve months following his injury, TM was referred to the *Be Clear Online* research study by the transitional rehabilitation service for ongoing dysarthria management. At this time, TM identified dysarthria as one of his greatest challenges, causing moderate frustration. Structural magnetic resonance imaging (MRI) revealed posterior fossa craniectomy with underlying bilateral cerebellar gliosis and encephalomalacia, secondary to bilateral cerebellar infarcts (see Figure 6.1). Pre-recruitment screening assessment revealed mild cognitive impairment on the Montreal Cognitive Assessment (MoCA = 24/30) (Nasreddine et al. 2005). Language was grossly intact with a score of 15/15 on the language screening test (Flamand-Roze et al. 2011).

Clinical findings

At the commencement of the *Be Clear Online* programme, TM was living alone, independently mobile, and able to manage his administrative affairs. He was participating in a home-based strength and balance programme under the supervision of an exercise physiologist and receiving community support for shopping and transportation when required. Prior to his injury, TM was an avid sportsman.

Initial informal assessment of TM's conversational speech revealed a moderate-to-severe reduction in speech intelligibility with a score of 6 based on an

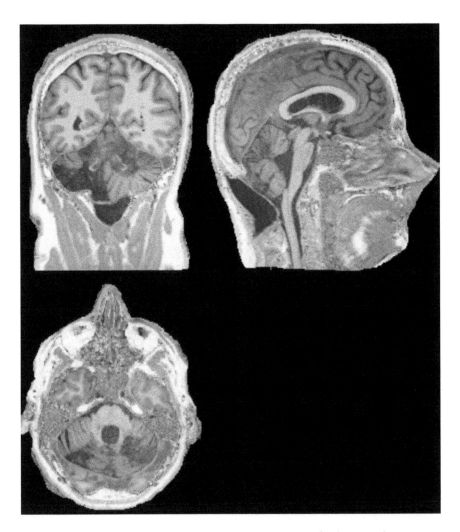

Figure 6.1 Structural MRI one week prior to commencement of online speech treatment

informal 7-point rating scale (0 = normal speech to 7 = severely unintelligible) (Darley, Aronson & Brown 1969). The presenting dysarthria was characterised by slow speech rate, excess and equal stress, articulatory imprecision, irregular articulatory breakdowns, mono-pitch, mono-loudness (with instances of excessive loudness variation), intermittent vocal strain, mild hypernasality, reduced respiratory control and shortened phrase length. These perceptual speech features together with lesion site were consistent with a diagnosis of ataxic-flaccid dysarthria (Figure 6.2).

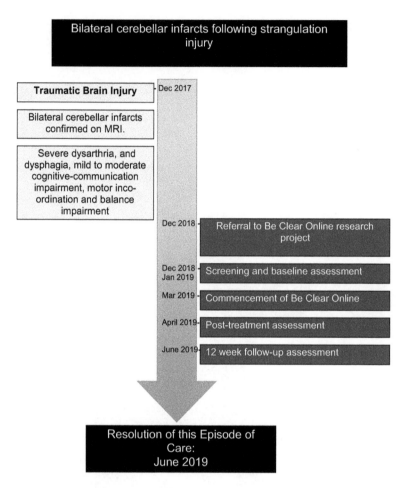

Figure 6.2 Timeline of episode of care

Assessment battery

Outcome measures were administered across three data collection intervals: (1) at baseline, (2) immediately post-treatment and (3) at follow-up (FUP) 12 weeks after treatment ended. Perceptual speech assessments and everyday communication measures were utilised to determine a baseline for speech intelligibility, perceived limitations on communication effectiveness and participation, and psychosocial impact of dysarthria. These assessments were conducted by an experienced SLP not directly involved in TM's online speech treatment. The outcome measures used included as follows: The AIDS (Yorkston & Beukelman 1984), the Communication Participation Item Bank (CPIB) (Baylor et al. 2012), the Communication Effectiveness Index-Modified (CETI-M) (Yorkston et al. 1999), the Dysarthria Impact Profile (DIP) (Walshe, Peach & Miller 2009) and paired comparison naive listener ratings of speech clarity (i.e. listeners were asked to indicate which speech sample they heard was clearer or easier to understand, sample A or B).

At the baseline assessment, TM achieved 79.5% sentence intelligibility on the AIDS, an overall speech rate of 88.34 words per minute (WPM), 69.91 intelligible words per minute (IWPM) and a communication efficiency ratio (CER) of 0.37 (see Table 6.1). These scores were calculated on averaged metrics across two testing sessions two days apart, to account for day-to-day variability in speech performance.

At baseline, TM achieved a total score of 17/30 on the 10-item short form of CPIB (see Table 6.1), with responses indicating his dysarthria interfered with participation across communicative contexts, either *'quite a bit'* (seven responses) or *'very much'* (three responses). TM and a familiar communication partner (i.e. close friend with regular social contact) identified substantial limitations in communication effectiveness on the CETI-M. TM self-rated his communication effectiveness a score of 27/70 and his communication partner, a score of 31/70. On a scale of 1 (*not at all effective*) to 7 (*very effective*), communication in eight out of ten possible scenarios was rated as 3 or below by both TM and his communication partner. TM reported his communication to be *not at all effective* in scenarios where he was required to speak on the phone.

A baseline total impact score (TIS) of 142/225 was achieved by TM on the DIP, indicating that his dysarthria was causing a negative impact upon his psychosocial well-being. Some examples of this adverse impact were reflected by TM's strong agreement that *'My speech has affected my life more than anything else'*, *'My speech problem has had a negative effect on how I see myself'* and *'When I speak I think I sound like somebody else, not me'*.

In addition to the measures mentioned earlier, audio recordings of a 40-second monologue on a topic of TM's choice were also obtained at each data collection point for the purpose of naïve listener paired comparison ratings of speech clarity. Ten naïve listeners (with no previous exposure to dysarthric speech) rated audio-recorded pre-treatment, post-treatment and FUP treatment speech samples. The samples were prepared in pairs for analysis in the following conditions: (1) pre-treatment versus post-treatment, (2) pre-treatment versus FUP, (3) post-treatment versus pre-treatment and (4) FUP versus pre-treatment. As per Park et al. (2016), the listeners were blinded to the assessment interval and instructed to indicate whether the first or second sample presented was 'clearer' or easier to understand, or whether there was no discernible difference.

Table 6.1 Be Clear Online speech outcomes

Assessment	Pre-treatment	Post-treatment	3 months post-treatment	Pre-post Percentage variation[a]	Pre-FUP Percentage variation
AIDS					
% sentence intelligibility	79.5	83.00	76.00	+4.40	-4.40
CER	0.37	0.44	0.39	+18.92	+5.45
WPM	88.34	98.25	97.42	+11.22	+10.27
IWPM	69.91	81.90	73.91	+17.15	+5.72
CETI-M					
Summary score speaker	27	48	54	+77.77	+100.00
Summary score caregiver	31	53	50	+70.97	+61.29
CPIB					
Total score	17	18	26	+5.88	+52.94
DIP					
TIS	142	157	154	+10.56	+8.45

Note: AIDS = Assessment of Intelligibility of Dysarthric Speech; % = percent; CER = communication efficiency ratio; WPM = words per minute; IWPM = intelligible words per minute, CETI-M = Communication Effectiveness Index- Modified; CPIB = Communication Participation Item Bank; DIP = Dysarthria Impact Profile; TIS = total impact score. [a] Percentage variation = post-treatment value – pre-treatment value/pre-treatment value) × 100

Therapeutic intervention

The *Be Clear Online* protocol aligned with the in-person protocol outlined by Park et al. (2016) in terms of programme structure, tasks and duration of treatment. The only exception was live demonstration of clear versus habitual speech by the treating clinician during the pre-practice session (as opposed to pre-recorded videos).

In order to determine appropriate technology for an online adaptation of this programme, a task analysis was conducted evaluating treatment tasks, types of interactions, stimuli, client responses required and necessary technical functions for online delivery (see Table 6.2). The analysis indicated that a synchronous videoconferencing platform with the capacity to share intervention materials (text and images) as well as audio capture with store-and-forward functionality, a whiteboard and end-to-end encryption (private and secure communication) was required.

A fit for purpose, readily available telehealth platform, Coviu (Coviu Global Pty Ltd) was selected for the *Be Clear Online* treatment programme. Coviu is a multi-device compatible, clinically validated telerehabilitation system with live videoconferencing and audio capture with store-and-forward functionality. For a 60-minute one-to-one call via Coviu, 9000-MB bandwidth was required, with a minimum upload and download requirement of 350 kbps. Coviu is typically accessed via a Wi-Fi-enabled device (e.g. tablet or computer). TM was provided with an Apple iPad (iOS, version 12.2) for the duration of the programme; however, he did not have access to Wi-Fi within his residence. This issue was addressed by using his mobile phone hotspot for treatment sessions, by voluntarily increasing his personal mobile plan at minimal cost for a period of one month.

TM consented to online treatment as part of the research study, which was delivered into his home by an experienced SLP. He received a 75-minute in-person training session (including the requisite pre-practice session) in his home prior to the commencement of intensive treatment, which included a live link to his treating clinician with opportunities to practice connection and experience online interaction and navigation of the Coviu platform, as well as clear speech stimulability testing. During this session, over-articulation was trialled and determined to be an effective strategy for TM to improve his speech intelligibility.

Following pre-practice, TM commenced the intensive phase of treatment involving one-hour sessions, four days per week, for a period of four weeks (total 16 sessions). Using the iPad, TM connected to each session via the Coviu App by accepting a call from his treating clinician. Once the call was accepted, TM was then asked to consent to the audio recording of speech samples during the session by touching the required response on the iPad screen. Individually tailored stimuli were prepared in digital format for uploading by the clinician during treatment sessions, and speech samples

Table 6.2 Be Clear: online task analysis

Phase	Components	Task	Interaction	Stimuli	Time	Client response	Technical function
Phase 1: Pre-Practice	Extended pre-practice	Shaping and instatement of clear speech concepts	Real time	Clinician examples of clear and unclear speech, text for reading, audio/verbal feedback on performance	60 minutes at outset of programme	Verbal rating of clear speech on scale (1–10)	VC, audio recording and playback, display text and whiteboard rating scale
Pre-Phase 2	Correspondence	Determining treatment target saliency	Asynchronous	List of everyday functional phrases and service requests out and about phrases	Unspecified	Written	Emails from clinician to client and from client to clinician
Phase 2: Intensive Practice	Pre-practice	Shaping and instatement of clear speech concepts using subset of session stimuli	Real time	Random presentation of subset of functional and out about phrases, reading aloud, picture description and conversation tasks	10 minutes	Verbal rating of clear speech on rating scale (1–10)	VC, display text and picture stimuli, audio recording and playback and whiteboard rating scale
Phase 2: Intensive Practice	Practice	Reading everyday functional phrases and out and about phrases	Real time	Text and audio/verbal feedback on performance	20 minutes	Verbal rating of clear speech on rating scale (1–10)	VC, display text, audio recording and playback and whiteboard rating scale

| Phase 2: Intensive Practice | Practice | Functional speech tasks: reading aloud, picture description and conversation | Real time | Text, picture stimuli and audio/verbal feedback on performance | 30 minutes | Verbal rating of clear speech on rating scale (1–10) | VC, display text and picture stimuli; audio recording and playback and whiteboard rating scale |
| Independent practice | Home Practice | Functional and out and about phrases, functional speech tasks, for example, using phone | Offline | Text | 15 minutes | Verbal | USB drive, recording device such as phone |

Note: VC = videoconferencing

were recorded throughout tasks and played back to TM for ratings of clarity via the audio capture with store-and-forward function in Coviu. Of note, once TM accepted the initial call to commence the session and consented to recording, the clinician maintained full control of the platform.

During the intensive treatment phase, TM was instructed to complete 15 minutes of daily self-managed home practice using his functional phrases, reading aloud, picture descriptions and transfer tasks. Voice Memos application (Apple Inc. 2018) was utilised during home practice, for TM to record his speech on the iPad during the relevant tasks and self-monitor speech clarity and modify where necessary. At the completion of the *Be Clear Online* programme, TM was instructed to maintain a daily practice schedule of ten minutes per day, three to five days per week, for a period of 12 weeks. TM completed the prescribed programme of 16 online sessions, daily self-managed home practice and 12 weeks of maintenance tasks following the completion of treatment. Treatment compliance in relation to home practice was corroborated during each treatment session, via a verbal check-in regarding chosen daily transfer tasks and the completion of other scheduled tasks. At the 12-week FUP assessment, TM confirmed that he had maintained the recommended home practice schedule.

Follow-up and outcomes

To provide a measure of the magnitude of change following treatment, percentage variation between pre- and post-speech treatment scores was calculated for each outcome measure (i.e. post-treatment value – pre-treatment value/pre-treatment value × 100) (see Table 6.1).

Perceptual outcomes

TM demonstrated a 4.4% increase in sentence intelligibility immediately post-treatment followed by a 4.4% decrease in sentence intelligibility at FUP. Neither of these fluctuations met the criterion of 8.6% for clinically significant change (Yorkston & Beukelman 1984). Post-treatment WPM increased by over 11%, IWPM increased by 17% and CER increased by approximately 19%. Although each of these scores remained above baseline levels at FUP, when compared to immediately post-treatment performance, a slight reduction in overall speech rate was observed (i.e. 0.84%), as well as a 9.74% reduction in CER and an 11.43% reduction in IWPM.

For the paired comparison speech sample ratings by naïve listeners, 80% of the ratings of the 20 pre-treatment/post-treatment comparisons indicated that post-treatment samples were clearer than pre-treatment samples. One rating (5%) indicated no discernible difference between pre- and post-treatment samples, and a further three ratings (15%) identified pre-treatment samples to be clearer than post-treatment samples. Of the 20 pre-treatment/FUP comparisons, 50%

of the ratings indicated that FUP samples were clearer than pre-treatment samples. One rating (5%) identified no discernible difference between pre-treatment and FUP samples, and nine ratings (45%) indicated that pre-treatment samples were clearer than FUP samples.

Everyday communication and psychosocial outcomes

In relation to ratings of communication effectiveness, TM achieved a 78% increase in his summary score on the CETI-M immediately post-treatment, which further increased by 100% at FUP (see Table 6.1). On a scale of 1 (*not at all effective*) to 7 (*very effective*), communication effectiveness in six out of ten possible scenarios was rated as 6 by TM, including speaking situations that involved the telephone. All other questions were assigned a rating of 4 or 5. Although lower in magnitude, TM's communication partner also reported overall post-treatment improvements in communication effectiveness, with increases of 71% immediately post-treatment and 61% at FUP.

Similar improvements in communication participation were reported by TM with increases in total scores on the CPIB of 5.88% (immediately post-treatment) and 52.94% (FUP) observed. Across most situations (i.e. six out of ten), TM reported his dysarthria to interfere with communication participation either '*not at all*' (two responses) or '*a little*' (four responses).

With respect to psychosocial outcomes, TM achieved an increase in total impact score on the DIP of 11% immediately post-treatment and 8.5% at FUP (see Table 6.1). This increase in score reflects a decrease in the psychosocial impact of dysarthria. TM reported at baseline that his dysarthria relative to other concerns was his greatest worry, followed by walking, eating, drinking and balance. At FUP, however, dysarthria had been relegated to fourth position on the concerns list.

Telepractice acceptability and feasibility

TM completed a satisfaction survey immediately post-treatment to evaluate perceptions of programme quality, effectiveness and convenience, as well as ease of telerehabilitation platform use and acceptance of online service delivery. TM *strongly agreed* that he could easily hear and see the SLP, that he felt comfortable communicating via the internet and that receiving online services was acceptable. He also *strongly agreed* that he would be happy to receive online services again; he was happy with the quality of the service; that online treatment was more convenient and saved travelling time. TM *agreed* that he needed assistance to use the telerehabilitation system, that his online treatment was effective and that he would prefer to receive treatment via the internet rather than in-person.

In summary, TM indicated a high level of satisfaction with the *Be Clear Online* speech treatment programme. Outcome measures also indicated post-treatment improvements on several rate-dependent intelligibility metrics, communication participation and effectiveness scores and psychosocial well-being.

Discussion

This case study demonstrated that the *Be Clear* programme can be successfully adapted and delivered online. The findings indicated a similar therapeutic effect to that achieved via in-person delivery (Park et al. 2016), with evidence of full treatment adherence, high treatment fidelity with the original programme and acceptable technical feasibility. A high level of satisfaction was also reported with online delivery of the programme.

Therapeutic effect

Increases in intelligibility metrics immediately post-treatment followed by decline at FUP suggest that acquisition of treatment behaviours was not retained over time. This phenomenon has been observed in other brain injury-focused dysarthria treatment studies (Wenke, Theodoros & Cornwell 2008), with the attenuation of motor speech performance being attributed to the blocked design of employed practice schedules (Knock et al. 2000). This theory lends some support to the current findings given that the *Be Clear* programme utilises a hybrid schedule of blocked and random practice. For example, the same individually tailored functional phrases are practiced in a block fashion in the first half of every session. During the second half of daily sessions, novel functional speech tasks (e.g. reading aloud, picture description and conversation) are practiced in a random manner. The attenuation of speech intelligibility over time within the current case may indicate that a hybrid treatment schedule enhances the acquisition of speech skills, but not long-term retention. An entirely random practice schedule may have facilitated the maintenance of improved speech intelligibility over time. Another hypothesis, however, may be that the observed instability in intelligibility may reflect the irregular nature of articulatory breakdown and prosodic abnormalities that are hallmark features of ataxic dysarthria (Duffy 2019). Despite these declines in post-treatment performance, all FUP AIDS scores except for sentence intelligibility remained above baseline and were considered to represent a positive therapeutic effect in relation to intelligible speech output produced within the context of increased speech rate.

The most substantial post-treatment changes were made in terms of self-reported communication effectiveness and participation, with stark improvements immediately post-treatment and continued increases at FUP on the CETI-M and CPIB. Post-treatment increases in communicative effectiveness were also corroborated by TM's communication partner. With respect to the psychosocial impact of dysarthria, relatively stable increases in total impact scores post-treatment on the DIP indicated a reduction in the perceived negative impact of dysarthria that was maintained over time. Increased communicative competence due to reduced instances of communication breakdown and subsequently the development of greater self-confidence in communicative interactions over time (Wenke, Theodoros & Cornwell 2008) may explain the upward trajectory of scores achieved on some outcome measures at FUP. Indeed, these findings support the concept of relationships between increased quality of life and successful communication participation (Tanner 2003).

The disparity between continued enhancement of communication effectiveness and participation ratings at FUP and reductions on intelligibility metrics may indicate that TM employed the clear speech strategy only when he determined that it was necessary (i.e. during functional communication exchanges as opposed to assessment contexts). Indeed, hyper-articulation theory implies that during over-articulated speech, speaker effort is increased so that listeners can better understand (Lindblom 1990). This maximal effort is accompanied by increases in timing, speed and distance of articulatory movements (Perkell 2012) and may not be able to be sustained continually.

Treatment adherence, fidelity and technical feasibility

To ensure treatment fidelity, technology that facilitated programme delivery in line with the original in-person *Be Clear* protocol was selected. All tasks, types of interactions, stimuli and client responses were consistent across delivery modes. Coviu enabled successful and easy delivery of treatment, as reported by TM and his treating clinician. Prior to commencement of the programme, the treating clinician received a two-hour training session targeting practice of the clear speech technique, *Be Clear* treatment schedule and how to use relevant applications on the Coviu platform. In addition, a fidelity examiner conducted a direct observation of one online treatment session and provided feedback to the clinician where required.

Coviu's design allowed the treating clinician to be in full technical control of the treatment session. Once the session commenced, TM was instructed in relation to tasks and required responses, with no further action required from him to engage with the Coviu platform. The initial task analysis identified the need for a whiteboard application on which treatment participants could physically mark ratings of speech clarity on a displayed scale, when played recorded audio samples. In practice, however, this application was not used with TM preferring to verbally state his rating. TM completed the prescribed programme online, attending all 16 treatment sessions and complied with home practice requirements.

The treating clinician maintained a log of technical difficulties. It was reported that audio and video quality was good, with occasional reductions in quality (e.g. freezing and pixilation). In one session, record and playback function did not work. These issues were typically resolved via the refresh function, computer restart or assistance from the Coviu help centre via online text chat.

As previously stated, training in the use of the technology is required for both clinicians and their clients. As part of this process, connectivity screening should be undertaken prior to accepting a client for online intervention. If connectivity is suboptimal and does not allow for treatment fidelity to be maintained, telepractice should not be implemented. Although Coviu is user-friendly, in-person training with Coviu was essential for seamless operation of the platform. In the pre-practice sessions for this case, live demonstrations of clear versus habitual speech were used instead of pre-recorded videos. Pre-recordings could be used, however, at the clinician's discretion if preferable, or needed in the event of variable connectivity.

Clinical considerations

Although the case study reported here was within the context of a research study, online delivery of the *Be Clear* speech treatment programme could be easily achieved within clinical settings. At the outset, time investment would be required for clinician training in the use of an appropriate telehealth platform. In most instances, platforms provide training manuals and/or online support that can facilitate self-directed training within a few hours. A patient training session (approximately half an hour to one hour) would also be required on how to interact with the platform during treatment sessions prior to commencement of the formal treatment program. As with all treatment approaches, patient suitability must be determined and should include stimulability for clear speech, adequate aided hearing and vision and cognitive capacity, stamina to engage in intensive treatment basic computer literacy and adequate internet connectivity. For some patients, support from an assistant in the home (e.g. family member or carer) during treatment sessions will be necessary. Clinicians must take into account their availability/case load allowance for intensive treatment (i.e. one-hour session four days per week for four weeks). Departing from the intensive treatment schedule is not recommended. The *Be Clear* programme applies principles of neuroplasticity in its design and requires adherence to an intensive treatment schedule. Delivery of the treatment could be shared between two clinicians, or alternatively with the assistance of trained and supervised students. If the patient or clinician is unable to commit to this level of treatment intensity, then an alternative treatment should be pursued.

In terms of required outcome measures, an abridged battery of the assessments reported in this chapter could be used clinically. At a minimum, a measure of speech intelligibility in conversation (using an informal rating scale) or paired comparison paradigm, together with a measure of communicative effectiveness and/or participation at baseline and post-treatment is recommended. At present, research evidence suggests that the *Be Clear* treatment programme can improve speech intelligibility and overall communicative function in adults with non-progressive dysarthria (Park et al. 2016). Evidence for the use of this programme with progressive dysarthria is currently unavailable; however, should a patient with dysarthria (regardless of aetiology) meet the abovementioned criteria, then the use of this technique with progressive conditions may be considered.

Satisfaction

The online programme provided a high level of satisfaction for TM. This case study suggests technologies that facilitate online delivery of rehabilitation programmes meet the needs of individuals with brain injury for effective and convenient treatment that fits within a complex schedule of competing priorities (Rietdijk et al. 2020). Indeed, TM stated that he preferred receiving online rather than in-person treatment as '*I could do it when I felt like, and I could do it at home*'.

Conclusion

The results presented within this case study demonstrate that in-person intensive dysarthria treatment programmes may be successfully adapted to the online environment with careful planning; appropriate technology selection and consideration of client attributes, training needs and level of support required. The positive therapeutic effect observed, and a high level of client satisfaction suggests that telepractice is a feasible mode of service delivery for dysarthria rehabilitation.

Key messages

- The *Be Clear* treatment programme can be successfully delivered online.
- A fit-for-purpose telehealth platform with audio store-and-forward functionality is essential.
- Application of principles of neuroplasticity in treatment design requires adherence to an intensive treatment schedule.
- Basic computer skills, internet connectivity, stimulability for clear speech and cognitive capacity must be considered for each patient prior to commencement of this program.

Acknowledgements

The authors thank TM and Jane Crombie (treating clinician) for their participation in the *Be Clear Online* pilot study and consenting to share multimedia materials for teaching and learning purposes. We would also like to acknowledge a team of participating investigators in the larger *Be Clear Online* research project: Louise Cahill, Atiyeh Vaezipour, Anna Farrell, Emma Finch, Adam Vogel, Stacie Park, Elizabeth Cardell and David Copland. We are grateful to the Motor Accident Insurance Commission (MAIC) of Queensland for funding this research.

References

Apple Inc. 2018, 'Voice Memos', [Mobile app]. Available at: App Store (Downloaded: 01 March 2018).

Baylor, C, Yorkston, K, Eadie, T, Kim, J, Chung, H & Amtmann, D 2012, 'The Communicative Participation Item Bank (CPIB): Item bank calibration and development of a disorder-generic form', *Journal of Speech, Language and Hearing Research*, vol. 56, pp. 1190–1208.

Beijer, LJ, Rietveld, TC, Hoskam, V, Geurts, AC & De Swart, BJ 2010a, 'Evaluating the feasibility and the potential efficacy of e-Learning-Based Speech Therapy (EST) as a web application for speech training in dysarthric patients with Parkinson's disease: A case study', *Telemedicine and e-Health*, vol. 16, pp. 732–738.

Beijer, LJ, Rietveld, TC, Van Beers, MM, Slangen, RM, Van Den Heuvel, H, De Swart, BJ & Geurts, AC 2010b, 'E-learning-based speech therapy: A web application for speech training', *Telemedicine and e-Health*, vol. 16, pp. 177–180.

Chan, MY, Chu, SY, Ahmad, K & Ibrahim, NM 2019, 'Voice therapy for Parkinson's disease via smartphone videoconference in Malaysia: A preliminary study', *Journal of Telemedicine and Telecare*, https://doi.org/10.1177/1357633X19870913

Constantinescu, G, Theodoros, D, Russell, T, Ward, E, Wilson, S & Wootton, R 2010, 'Assessing disordered speech and voice in Parkinson's disease: A telerehabilitation application', *International Journal of Language & Communication Disorders*, vol. 45, pp. 630–644.

Constantinescu, G, Theodoros, D, Russell, T, Ward, E, Wilson, S & Wootton, R 2011, 'Treating disordered speech and voice in Parkinson's disease online: A randomized controlled non-inferiority trial', *International Journal of Language & Communication Disorders*, vol. 46, pp. 1–16.

Covert, LT, Slevin, JT & Hatterman, J 2018, 'The effect of telerehabilitation on missed appointment rates', *International Journal of Telerehabilitation*, vol. 10, no. 2, pp. 65–72.

Darley, FL, Aronson, AE & Brown, JR 1969, 'Differential diagnostic patterns of dysarthria', *Journal of Speech and Hearing Research*, vol. 12, pp. 246–269.

Dias, AE, Limongi, JCP, Barbosa, ER & Hsing, WT 2016, 'Voice telerehabilitation in Parkinson's disease', *CoDAS*, vol. 28, no. 2, pp. 176–181.

Duffy, J 2019, *Motor speech disorders: Substrates, differential diagnosis, and management*, 4th edn, Elsevier, St Louis, MO.

Duffy, JR, Werven, GW & Aronson, AE 1997, 'Telemedicine and the diagnosis of speech and language disorders', *Mayo Clinic Proceedings*, vol. 72, pp. 1116–1122.

Enderby, P 1983, *Frenchay dysarthria assessment*, College-Hill Press, San Diego, CA.

Feeney, MP, Xu, Y, Surface, M, Shah, H, Vanegas-Arroyave, N, Chan, AK, Delaney, E, Przedborski, S, Beck, JC & Alcalay, RN 2021, 'The impact of COVID-19 and social distancing on people with Parkinson's disease: A survey study', *NPJ Parkinson's Disease*, vol. 7, no. 1, p. 10.

Flamand-Roze, C, Falissard, B, Roze, E, Maintigneux, L, Beziz, J, Chacon, A, Join-Lambert, C, Adams, D & Denier, C 2011, 'Validation of a new language screening tool for patients with acute stroke: The Language Screening Test (LAST)', *Stroke*, vol. 42, pp. 1224–1229.

Fong, R, Tsai, CF & Yiu, OY 2021, 'The implementation of telepractice in speech language pathology in Hong Kong during the COVID-19 pandemic', *Telemedicine and e-Health*, vol. 27, pp. 30–38.

Griffin, M, Bentley, J, Shanks, J & Wood, C 2018, 'The effectiveness of Lee Silverman Voice Treatment therapy issued interactively through an iPad device: A non-inferiority study', *Journal of Telemedicine and Telecare*, vol. 24, pp. 209–215.

Hill, AJ, Theodoros, DG, Russell, TG, Cahill, LM, Ward, EC & Clark, KM 2006, 'An internet-based telerehabilitation system for the assessment of motor speech disorders: A pilot study', *American Journal of Speech-Language Pathology*, vol. 15, pp. 45–56.

Hill, AJ, Theodoros, DG, Russell, TG & Ward, EC 2009, 'The redesign and re-evaluation of an internet-based telerehabilitation system for the assessment of dysarthria in adults', *Telemedicine and e-Health*, vol. 15, pp. 840–850.

Howell, S, Tripoliti, E & Pring, T 2009, 'Delivering the Lee Silverman Voice Treatment (LSVT) by web camera: A feasibility study', *International Journal of Language & Communication Disorders*, vol. 44, pp. 287–300.

Knock, T, Ballard, K, Robin, D & Schmidt, R 2000, 'Influence of order of stimulus presentation on speech motor learning: A principled approach to treatment for apraxia of speech', *Aphasiology*, vol. 14, pp. 653–668.

Lindblom, B 1990, 'Explaining phonetic variation: A sketch of the H & H theory', in Hardcastle, WJ & Marchal, A (eds.), *Speech production and speech modelling*, Kluwer Academic, Dordrecht, the Netherlands.

Nasreddine, Z, Philllips, N, Bédirian, V, Charbonneau, S, Whitehead, V, Collin, I, Cummings, JL & Chertkow, H 2005, 'The Montreal Cognitive Assessment (MoCA): A brief screening tool for mild cognitive impairment', *Journal of the American Geriatrics Society*, vol. 53, pp. 695–699.

Park, S, Theodoros, D, Finch, E & Cardell, E 2016, 'Be clear: A new intensive speech treatment for adults with nonprogressive dysarthria', *American Journal of Speech-Language Pathology*, vol. 25, pp. 97–110.

Perkell, JS 2012, 'Movement goals and feedback and feedforward control mechanisms in speech production', *Journal of Neurolinguistics*, vol. 25, pp. 382–407.

Quinn, R, Park, S, Theodoros, D & Hill, AJ 2019, 'Delivering group speech maintenance therapy via telerehabilitation to people with Parkinson's disease: A pilot study', *International Journal of Speech-Language Pathology*, vol. 21, pp. 385–394.

Ramig, LO, Sapir, S, Fox, C & Countryman, S 2001, 'Changes in vocal loudness following intensive voice treatment (LSVT*) in individuals with Parkinson's disease: A comparison with untreated patients and normal age-matched controls', *Movement Disorders*, vol. 16, pp. 79–83.

Rietdijk, R, Power, E, Attard, M & Togher, L 2020, 'Acceptability of telehealth-delivered rehabilitation: Experiences and perspectives of people with traumatic brain injury and their carers', *Journal of Telemedicine & Telecare*, https://doi.org/10.1177/1357633X20923824

Saiyed, M, Hill, AJ, Russell, TG, Theodoros, DG & Scuffham, P 2020, 'Cost analysis of home telerehabilitation for speech treatment in people with Parkinson's disease', *Journal of Telemedicine and Telecare*, https://dx.doi.org/10.1177/1357633X20948302

Speech Pathology Australia 2014, *Telepractice in speech pathology*, viewed February 19, www.speechpathologyaustralia.org.au/SPAweb/Members/Position_Statements/SPAweb/Members/Position_Statements/Position_Statements.aspx?hkey=b1a46941-246c-4609-bacc-1c1b5c52d19d

Tanner, D 2003, *The psychology of neurogenic communication disorders: A primer for health care professionals*, Allyn & Bacon, Boston, MA.

Theodoros, DG, Hill, AJ & Russell, TG 2016, 'Clinical and quality of life outcomes of speech treatment for Parkinson's disease delivered to the home via telerehabilitation: A noninferiority randomized controlled trial', *American Journal of Speech-Language Pathology*, vol. 25, pp. 214–232.

Theodoros, DG, Russell, TG, Hill, A, Cahill, L & Clark, K 2003, 'Assessment of motor speech disorders online: A pilot study', *Journal of Telemedicine and Telecare*, vol. 9, no. 2_suppl, pp. 66–68.

Walshe, M, Peach, RK & Miller, N 2009, 'Dysarthria impact profile: Development of a scale to measure psychosocial effects', *International Journal of Language & Communication Disorders*, vol. 44, pp. 693–715.

Wenke, RJ, Theodoros, D & Cornwell, P 2008, 'The short- and long-term effectiveness of the LSVT® for dysarthria following TBI and stroke', *Brain Injury*, vol. 22, pp. 339–352.

Yorkston, KM & Beukelman, DR 1984, *Assessment of intelligibility of dysarthric speech*, Pro-Ed, Austin, TX.

Yorkston, KM, Beukelman, DR, Strand, EA & Bell, KR 1999, *Management of motor speech disorders in children and adults*, 2nd edn, Pro-Ed, Austin, TX.

Chapter 7

Looking beyond the impairment

The psychosocial impact of dysarthria on the speaker

Margaret Walshe

Introduction

This chapter is concerned with the psychosocial impact of dysarthria from the speaker's perspective. This man (TS) has Friedreich's ataxia (FRDA), which is an autosomal recessive progressive neurodegenerative disease affecting the central and peripheral nervous systems. It is also associated with non-neurological symptoms such as scoliosis and cardiomyopathy. It is the most common inherited ataxia in Europe with prevalence showing large regional differences, between south-west Europe (1 in 20,000) and the north and east of Europe (1 in 25,000) (Vankan, 2013). It is typically diagnosed in the first or second decade of life, but it can, as in this case report, be diagnosed later. Late onset FRDA occurs in people aged 25–39 years (Fearon et al., 2020). It is likely that TS had signs and symptoms at age 28 years that were associated with FRDA. People with late onset FRDA are likely to have a milder, more slowly evolving disease than people diagnosed in the first and in the earlier second decades (Bhidayasiri et al., 2005; Indelicato et al., 2020).

In FRDA, the cerebellum, brainstem and the spinal cord are affected resulting in an ataxic gait. Visual disorders may also be present as well as sensorineural deafness, cognitive impairment and dysarthria. Dysarthria is one of the key diagnostic signs in FRDA. It is usually a mixed ataxic/spastic/flaccid type dysarthria due to the systems other than the cerebellum being affected. Blaney and Hewlett (2007) along with Folker et al. (2010) have examined the perceptual characteristics of dysarthria associated with FRDA. Folker et al. suggest that there are three subgroups of dysarthria presentations in FRDA: those with (a) mild dysarthria symptoms, (b) increased velopharyngeal involvement and (c) increased laryngeal dysfunction.

Dysarthria transcends the physiological impairment to impact identity, self-concept and self-esteem that, in turn, affect social participation and quality of life. This is clear from qualitative research with people with dysarthria associated with a number of different aetiologies (Brady et al., 2011; Dickson et al., 2008; Gillivan Murphy et al., 2019; Miller et al., 2008; Walshe & Miller,

DOI: 10.4324/9781003172536-7

2011). The experience of living with dysarthria is also highly individual, and this must be considered in the approach to assessment and intervention.

Case report

At the time of this therapy episode, TS was a 38-year-old man who was married with four children, the youngest being eight years old. Ten years earlier, he developed left lower limb ataxia and limb weakness with mild dysarthria a year later. He presented to the speech and language therapy outpatient clinic five years after that with a mild dysarthria that he attributed to medication, although this was ruled out. His medical diagnosis was possible spinocerebellar degeneration. Therapy focused on oro-motor exercises and decreasing speech rate. TS had not found therapy helpful and discontinued attending. He continued to work as a baker, and the aetiology of the motor and speech impairment remained under investigation. There was a family history of neurological difficulties. His mother had developed ataxia and dysarthria at 44 years of age, and his sister had a history of 'unsteadiness' beginning at 35 years of age. His mother was now deceased.

In this episode of therapy, he contacted the speech and language therapist (SLT) at the request of the neurologist. His dysarthria seemed to be increasing in severity. He complained of increased fatigue and unsteadiness in his feet. FRDA was recently diagnosed, and TS was coping with this diagnosis and its implications for his young family.

Presenting concerns

TS attended the clinic for the first session alone. His main concern at this initial visit was the perceptual quality of his speech, the trajectory of the disease and his resolve to find a different role for himself through seeking new employment. His children were young, and he was keen to financially support the family. He was concerned that his chances of obtaining employment would be reduced because of his dysarthria. He worried that people would think he had been drinking because his speech was slurred and that unfamiliar listeners would think he had some cognitive impairment and would judge him negatively.

Clinical findings

TS walked unaided with an ataxic gait. He had attended occupational therapy previously, and his home had been adapted with some handrails to decrease his risk of falling. He reported no visual or hearing difficulties. His speech was perceptually an ataxic type of dysarthria with intelligible comprehensible speech.

Diagnostic focus and assessment

An assessment of intelligibility of TS's dysarthria on the Assessment of Intelligibility of Dysarthric Speech (AIDS) (Yorkston & Beukelman, 1981) indicated a score of 95% at sentence level and 98% at word level. The severity of dysarthria using an adaptation Yorkston et al.'s Dysarthria Rating of Severity Scale (Donovan et al., 2008) was rated at Stage 2: *Obvious speech disorder with intelligible speech*. He had changes in voice, reduced loudness, reduced pitch variability and had difficulty making himself understood in noisy environments. During the assessment, it was clear that TS was aware of the strategies to help improve intelligibility such as decreasing speech rate, alternating stress on words but he was not always comfortable using these strategies as he believed that they were unhelpful particularly with strangers.

On the Communication Effectiveness Survey (CES) (Donovan et al., 2008), where TS was asked to rate how effective his speech was in different communication situations, he scored 15/32. TS described difficulty speaking in particular communication contexts, specifically when he was anxious, when he had to speak through a glass screen and when he was in a noisy environment. In discussing the CES responses with TS, it was apparent that a lot of his communication difficulties arose because of a lack of confidence and a perception that listeners were evaluating him on the basis of his dysarthria. TS was very self-conscious about his speech and had decreased his level of participation with friends.

The Dysarthria Impact Profile (DIP) (Walshe et al., 2009) (Table 7.1) was administered to examine the impact of his dysarthria and to help target goals for therapy. Each statement in the DIP elicits a score ranging from 1 (most negative impact) to 5 (least negative impact). The possible range of scores from all statements in the first four sections of the DIP is from 48 to 240. Scores from 48 to 96 are considered low scores as they imply that respondents have received an average score of either one or two for each statement. Similarly, a score between 192 and 240 is considered high, with people receiving an average rating of four or five for each statement. The overall impact score for TS was 117 suggesting that dysarthria had a considerable negative impact of his life. The mean scores for each of the first four sections were then calculated. This allowed for broad comparison across sections (Table 7.1). The section with the lowest score (most negative impact) was Section C 'How I feel Others React to My Speech' although the other sections also received low scores.

The final section of the DIP (Section E) asks the person to list four things, apart from speech and communication, that upset or worry them. TS listed that he was most concerned or worried about passing FRDA onto his children. He was also worried about his walking. His worry about his speech came after both these items. This section of the DIP was useful as it helped place dysarthria in context of the condition in which it exists.

Table 7.1 Assessment timepoint 1: TS's scores on dysarthria impact profile (Walshe et al., 2009)

Sub-section of DIP	Score
Section A: The effect of dysarthria on me as a person	Total score: 33 (mean score: 2.75)
Section B: Accepting my dysarthria	Total score: 24 (mean score: 2.40)
Section C: How I feel others react to my speech	Total score: 32 (mean score: 2.28)
Section D: How dysarthria affects my communication with others	Total score: 28 (mean score: 2.33)
	Total DIP score: 117
Section E: Dysarthria relative to other worries and concerns	3 (something that he is concerned/ worried about)

Sections A and B of the DIP explore 'The effect of dysarthria on me as a person' and 'Accepting my dysarthria', respectively. To explore these further, a semantic differential scale, amended from that used by Tyerman and Humphrey (1984) for people with acquired dysarthria (Miller et al., 2011; Walshe, 2003), was also administered. This semantic differential scale was originally developed to measure change in self-concept and psychological state after traumatic brain injury. The scale comprises 20 bipolar adjectives, alternated to minimise the risk of people responding on one direction of the scale. Adjective pairs are rated on a 7-point scale from 1 (negative pole) to 7 (positive pole). People are asked to rate 'Present Self' (self in the last two weeks); 'Past Self' (self in the six months prior to the onset of dysarthria) and 'Future Self' (expectations a year into the future). TS rated Past Self, Present Self and Future Self. He scored 127 overall on constructs that relate to Past Self. Low scores being more negative. He scored 71 on constructs that related to Present Self and 95 for constructs that relate to Future Self. There was no change between Past, Present and Future Self on three constructs. TS still saw himself as friendly, intelligent and caring and anticipated that he would remain so in the future. The greatest change between Past Self and Present Self were in four constructs where TS saw himself as much more self-conscious, dissatisfied, unhappy and more irritable that he was prior to becoming dysarthric. His Future Self scores saw the greatest change in being more in control, less self-conscious, more self-confident, feeling more of value, being less irritable and being more patient. These scores suggest that TS was optimistic about the future while also remaining realistic – he did not envisage a return to his 'Past Self'.

At the end of the assessment, the clinical hypothesis was that whilst TS's speech was mildly dysarthric with high levels of speech intelligibility and comprehensibility, dysarthria had impacted on his self-concept and self-esteem. He perceived that listeners, particularly strangers, evaluated him negatively because of his speech and this impacted on his social participation.

Therapeutic focus and assessment

TS was seen at home as part of a trial domiciliary outreach service for the hospital department. This enabled observation of TS communicating in his home environment, helped establish a relationship with TS's wife who couldn't always come to the clinic and to observe the communication facilitators and barriers to communication in his own home. It was a busy but friendly home. The support from his family was obvious, and he took an active role in parenting. It was decided to trial a series of six sessions over a seven-week period with a review at the end of this time. The agreed focus of therapy was to explore the effect that dysarthria had on TS directly and to collaboratively examine ways in which this could be improved.

With his consent, TS's wife took part in the initial session where the results of the DIP and the semantic differential scale were explored. TS believed that he had accepted his dysarthria despite the DIP scores but that the uncertainty regarding further speech deterioration in the future resulted in lower scores in this section. It was agreed that Sections C and D of the DIP were closely linked – TS's perception of other people's reaction impacted on his communication.

It was suggested that through tackling other people's response to speech and educating listeners that TS might gain more confidence in communication situations. An outline of the intervention programme is provided in Table 7.2. A key focus was TS's self-management of his dysarthria. This involved problem-solving, decision-making, identifying resources and re-interpreting situations (see Baylor & Darling-White, 2020; Yorkston et al., 2017 for a further discussion on participation focused intervention and self-management of dysarthria).

In our therapy sessions, we discovered that integral to TS's own self-concept and self-esteem was his own construing of people with speech impairment in the past and in his childhood. This was a valuable discussion that led to the importance of educating people about dysarthria – a role that TS was happy to consider in the future.

Follow-up and outcomes

TS was reviewed again six months after the last therapy session (Figure 7.1: Timeline). This time he was seen in the clinic setting. He had not completed the computer training due to problems with double vision but was enjoying his role as 'house husband'. The CES was re-administered with an improved in

Table 7.2 TS's Intervention programme

Sessions 1–3. Listener reactions	Agreed strategy	Outcome
Being ignored in conversation. TS cited an incident earlier in the first therapy week where a family member had asked, 'How is he?' in TS's presence. TS discussed the impact of that incident openly and the effect of those conversations on his self-esteem.	TS's wife agreed to tackle those situations by reverting to TS and discouraging these types of conversations.	This was an ongoing project with TS's brother and father also providing support here.
Speaking to strangers on the phone. TS found this situation difficult, and people often hung up on the phone once he commenced talking. He believed that this was because he sounded intoxicated.	TS would start the call stating that he had a speech problem and asking the listener to be patient. He trialled this strategy daily by requesting information from local services and department stores. He recorded and gave feedback on listener reaction.	TS was uncomfortable with this initially but found that listeners responded more patiently and positively.
Speaking to people in his children's school. TS did not speak to other parents in the school playground, as he did not want them to think he had been 'drinking because of his speech'. He also did not attend parent–teacher meetings for the same reason.	When waiting to pick up his children outside the classroom, he agreed to arrive early and start a conversation stating that he had a speech problem, if the opportunity and timing was right. He agreed to meet with teachers informally to help with confidence in larger meetings.	This took a little while, but TS realised that the other parents were already aware of his condition and that his speech problem was associated with his condition.
Asking for items in shops. TS shopped in supermarkets where he did not have to talk to strangers unless he could not find an item. He found places such as small newspaper outlets and post offices difficult.	We agreed that TS would take a list of what he needed and if the listener was unable to understand him, he would present this note. That would provide TS with some security in these situations. TS would also tell the listener that he had a problem with his speech.	TS found this useful. The list was a source of re-assurance, and he would only use this if his speech was not intelligible.

(Continued)

Table 7.2 (Continued)

Sessions 3–4. Managing the impairment	Agreed strategy	Outcome
Fatigue. TS recognised that fatigue impacted on his speech. He tended to push past this fatigue and not give in. The need for rest was discussed.	TS kept a diary of when his speech was more prone to fatigue. This generally followed a pattern and was dependent on other activities that day. TS timed visits to his father and wider family more carefully around this.	TS believed that this helped give him some control over his dysarthria.

Sessions 1–6. Living with dysarthria	Agreed strategy	Outcome
This topic was covered in all sessions but became a stronger focus in the last three sessions.	**It was agreed to focus on 'abilities'** with a plan to learn new computer skills with aids and adaptations. TS was linked in with community supports to help with keyboard skills and an occupational therapist to help with an adapted keyboard and computer monitor. **TS's role in the home:** TS's identity as 'breadwinner' was challenged when he became unemployed. He believed this was central to his self-esteem. With TS's wife, we problem-solved TS's need to discover a new role within the family unit with clear responsibility for household tasks and chores.	TS had already informally taken on more of a role within the home. This clarity in role with open discussion within the family helped TS transition into this new role.

scores to 19/32. This improvement was mainly due to change in speaking to strangers on the phone. The semantic differential scale was re-administered. TS could see his scores from the previous session while completing this and was able to comment more reliably on what had changed. There was a slight increase in scores overall. Present Self was re-scored. TS continued to see himself as caring, friendly and intelligent and scored 77 (an increase in six points from the first assessment) with only minor changes across constructs. Future Self was not re-scored as TS was upset that his mobility and vision were

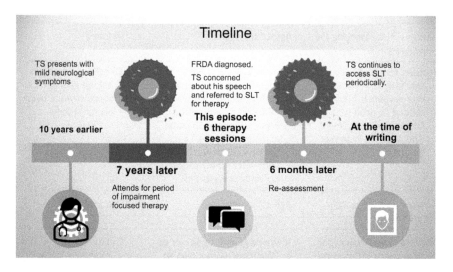

Figure 7.1 Timeline

changing, and he had new fears about the future. These changes may also have been reflected in the scores of Present Self.

The DIP was also re-administered (Table 7.3). Again, TS could see his scores from the previous session. He reported that he now believed his communication was more effective when talking to strangers on the phone and having a conversation with someone at a distance as he was using more strategies to help the listener. His overall scores on the DIP had increased from 117 to 148; the greatest change being in Sections A and D (Tables 7.1 and 7.3). In the intervening six months, TS reported that he was increasingly

Table 7.3 Assessment timepoint 2: TS's scores on dysarthria impact profile (Walshe et al., 2009)

Sub-section of DIP	Score
Section A: The effect of dysarthria on me as a person	Total score: 42 (mean score: 3.50)
Section B: Accepting my dysarthria	Total score: 28 (mean score: 2.80)
Section C: How I feel others react to my speech	Total score: 37 (mean score: 2.64)
Section D: How dysarthria affects my communication with others	Total score: 41 (mean score: 3.41)
	Total DIP score: 148
Section E: Dysarthria relative to other worries and concerns	4 (something that he is slightly concerned/worried about)

concerned about his walking as he felt more unsteady on his feet. TS believed that the most important part of speech and language therapy in this most recent episode was the opportunity to focus on its impact and to problem-solve situations. He did not believe he could do that within his family or with friends, as he did not wish to 'burden' them. He was mindful that his medical condition impacted everyone that was close to him. The hereditary nature of FRDA also concerned him.

TS suggested that therapy in his home was more helpful in building a rapport that provided a solid basis for exploring emotional issues beyond impairment. Of course, this relationship is also important in the longer term as TS's dysarthria progresses, and the focus of therapy shifts again to increasing speech intelligibility.

Discussion

There are many important lessons from this case report. First, the link between impairment and psychosocial impact is not linear. TS had very good speech intelligibility. His intelligibility scores are similar to the ratings amongst participants in Blayney and Hewlett's study where they examined the characteristics of dysarthria amongst a group of speakers with FRDA. He may, therefore, not be seen as a priority for speech and language therapy in some hard-pressed services. The impairment-focused therapy that he did receive focused on strategies that he argued made his speech sound different – slowing rate, altering prosodic elements, etc. Yet, it was the perceptual characteristics of his speech that impacted his self-confidence in participation the most. People with progressive neurodegenerative dysarthria want more than an impairment-based approach (Atkinson-Clement et al., 2019; Walshe, 2003; Yorkston et al., 2017), especially when the gradual deterioration in intelligibility may stretch over many years before intensive, focused work on articulation is required but where repercussions for self-esteem and self-image may already be exercising a considerable effect.

Of course, it is frequently argued that an impairment-focused therapy might indirectly result in increased confidence in social interactions (Bryans et al., 2021). Lowit et al. (2020) describe the use of a modified version of LSVT LOUD (r) with people with FRDA. Participant reports in interviews after the intervention suggest some positive effects of the impairment-focused treatment on confidence and social participation. However, one cannot always expect that an impairment-based approach will impact on psychological and social functioning (Gillivan-Murphy et al., 2019). TS had impairment-focused therapy in the past that did not alleviate his anxiety around social situations. In this instance, a less impairment-focused approach resulted in considerable gains in participation.

Second, completing the non-impairment-focused assessments such as the DIP, CES and semantic differential scale were invaluable in directing therapy.

Individuals with dysarthria can change their perception of themselves as communicators over time in these progressive neurological conditions (Miller et al., 2011). Changes do not relate straightforwardly to other clinical measures. Major impact can occur despite good intelligibility levels. Exploring self-perceptions, individual reactions and coping strategies are argued to be a vital part of assessment and management (see Chapter 1).

The assessments used in this case report not only provided insight into how dysarthria had impacted TS but also served as a point for discussion and an opportunity to provide possible solutions to difficulties. Employing the DIP, CES and semantic differential scale, as well as other similar scales also helped identify situational/interaction variables that can be a useful pointer in any impairment-focused therapy approach. They also allowed impairment-based approaches taught in other therapy episodes to be consolidated into TS's communication interactions.

The DIP scores suggested that the psychosocial impact had decreased somewhat for TS, and whilst the clinically meaningful difference in test scores is not established for this test, the positive change in TS's attitude towards communication situations suggests that the changes in scores are clinically relevant. The increase in scores in the semantic differential scale was small, but no major changes here were anticipated, as no psychological therapies were provided. One might question at this point if more psychological interventions delivered by trained clinicians would be helpful. Access to psychological services tend to be reserved for the people who are more significantly impacted psychologically by their condition. The impact of dysarthria on social participation was only truly exposed by discussion and assessments. Outwardly, it appeared that TS was coping with his condition. The need for psychological support for people with neurodegenerative diseases including FRDA is considerable (Simpson et al., 2021), and a team approach to dysarthria management is important.

Third, in progressive neurological disease such as FRDA, the changing context in which dysarthria exists must always be considered. Section E of the DIP showed that whilst TS was anxious about his speech, there were also equally pressing worries and concerns, unrelated to speech. The impact of dysarthria on the speaker is highly individual (Walshe & Miller, 2011), and although factors such as age of onset, length of time living with dysarthria and its underlying condition as well as dysarthria profile play a role, it is clear that common themes exist and that treating dysarthria in isolation is not ideal (see Chapter 1).

Finally, providing TS with the opportunity to talk about his dysarthria and in his everyday communication environment was invaluable, and its influence in outcomes cannot be underestimated. In Dickson et al.'s study with people with dysarthria post-stroke, people commented that they would have liked SLTs to visit them at home (Dickson et al., 2008). It is not always possible to see people in their own homes, not would many people want it, but it was mutually beneficial in this instance.

TS continues to access SLT periodically. Some items are changed to protect his anonymity. He consented to provide this information, which was part of a larger clinical service initiative.

Key messages

- The psychosocial impact of dysarthria can have considerable impact on the speaker and their family.
- The impact of dysarthria can be disproportionate to the severity of the physiological impairment.
- Assessment of psychosocial impact should be an integral part of evaluation, and intervention programmes should consider psychological and social consequences of dysarthria when developing therapeutic goals.
- Exploring the impact of dysarthria on the speaker with key strategies to help people live with their dysarthria should be a central focus of therapy.

References

Atkinson-Clement, C., Letanneux, A., Baille, G., Cuartero, M. C., Véron-Delor, L., Robieux, C., Berthelot, M., Robert, D., Azulay, J. P., Defebvre, L., Ferreira, J., Eusebio, A., Moreau, C., & Pinto, S. (2019). Psychosocial impact of dysarthria: The patient-reported outcome as part of the clinical management. *Neurodegenerative Diseases*, 19(1), 12–21.

Baylor, C., & Darling-White, M. (2020). Achieving participation-focused intervention through shared decision making: Proposal of an age- and disorder-generic framework. *American Journal of Speech-Language Pathology*, 29(3), 1335–1360.

Bhidayasiri, R., Perlman, S. L., Pulst, S. M., & Geschwind, D. H. (2005). Late-onset Friedreich ataxia: Phenotypic analysis, magnetic resonance imaging findings, and review of the literature. *Archives of Neurology*, 62(12), 1865–1869. https://doi.org/10.1001/archneur.62.12.1865

Blaney, B., & Hewlett, N. (2007). Dysarthria and Friedreich's ataxia: What can intelligibility assessment tell us? *International Journal of Language & Communication Disorders*, 42(1), 19–37.

Brady, M. C., Clark, A. M., Dickson, S., Paton, G., & Barbour, R. S. (2011). The impact of stroke-related dysarthria on social participation and implications for rehabilitation. *Disability and Rehabilitation*, 33(3), 178–186.

Bryans, L. A., Palmer, A. D., Anderson, S., Schindler, J., & Graville, D. J. (2021). The impact of Lee Silverman Voice Treatment (LSVT LOUD®) on voice, communication, and participation: Findings from a prospective, longitudinal study. *Journal of Communication Disorders*, 89, 106031.

Dickson, S., Barbour, R. S., Brady, M., Clark, A. M., & Paton, G. (2008). Patients' experiences of disruptions associated with post-stroke dysarthria. *International Journal of Language & Communication Disorders*, 43(2), 135–153. https://doi.org/10.1080/13682820701862228.

Donovan, N. J., Kendall, D. L., Young, M. E., & Rosenbek, J. C. (2008). The communicative effectiveness survey: Preliminary evidence of construct validity. *American Journal of Speech-Language Pathology*, 17(4), 335–347.

Fearon, C., Lonergan, R., Ferguson, D., Byrne, S., Bradley, D., Langan, Y., & Redmond, J. (2020). Very-late-onset Friedreich's ataxia: Diagnosis in a kindred with late-onset cerebellar ataxia. *Practical Neurology*, 20(1), 55–58.

Folker, J., Murdoch, B., Cahill, L., Delatycki, M., Corben, L., & Vogel, A. (2010). Dysarthria in Friedreich's ataxia: A perceptual analysis. *Folia Phoniatrica et Logopaedica*, 62(3), 97–103.

Gillivan-Murphy, P., Miller, N., & Carding, P. (2019). Voice treatment in Parkinson's disease: Patient perspectives. *Research and Reviews in Parkinsonism*, 9, 29–42.

Indelicato, E., Nachbauer, W., Eigentler, A., Amprosi, M., Matteucci Gothe, R., Giunti, P., Mariotti, C., Arpa, J., Durr, A., Klopstock, T., Schöls, L., Giordano, I., Bürk, K., Pandolfo, M., Didszdun, C., Schulz, J. B., Boesch, S., & EFACTS (European Friedreich's Ataxia Consortium for Translational Studies) (2020). Onset features and time to diagnosis in Friedreich's Ataxia. *Orphanet Journal of Rare Diseases*, 15(1), 198.

Lowit, A., Egan, A., & Hadjivassiliou, M. (2020). Feasibility and acceptability of Lee Silverman Voice Treatment in progressive ataxias. *Cerebellum* (London, England), 19(5), 701–714.

Miller, N., Noble, E., Jones, D., Allcock, L., & Burn, D. J. (2008). How do I sound to me? Perceived changes in communication in Parkinson's disease. *Clinical Rehabilitation*, 22(1), 14–22.

Miller, N., Andrew, S., Noble, E., & Walshe, M. (2011). Changing perceptions of self as a communicator in Parkinson's disease: A longitudinal follow-up study. *Disability and Rehabilitation*, 33(3), 204–210.

Simpson, J., Eccles, F., & Zarotti, N. (2021). *Psychological interventions for people with Huntington's disease, Parkinson's disease, motor neurone disease and multiple sclerosis: Evidence based guidance*. Leicester: The British Psychological Society.

Tyerman, A., & Humphrey, M. (1984). Changes in self-concept following severe head injury. *International Journal of Rehabilitation Research. Internationale Zeitschrift fur Rehabilitationsforschung. Revue internationale de recherches de readaptation*, 7(1), 11–23.

Vankan, P. (2013). Prevalence gradients of Friedreich's ataxia and R1b haplotype in Europe co-localize, suggesting a common Palaeolithic origin in the Franco-Cantabrian ice age refuge. *Journal of Neurochemistry*, 126(1), 11–20.

Walshe, M. (2003). *'You have no idea: You have no idea what it is like . . . not to be able to talk': Exploring the impact and experience of acquired neurological dysarthria from the speaker's perspective*. PhD Thesis. Trinity College Dublin, Ireland.

Walshe, M., Peach, R. K., & Miller, N. (2009). Dysarthria impact profile: Development of a scale to measure psychosocial effects. *International Journal of Language & Communication Disorders*, 44(5), 693–715.

Walshe, M., & Miller, N. (2011). Living with acquired dysarthria: The speaker's perspective. *Disability and Rehabilitation*, 33(3), 195–203.

Yorkston, K., & Beukelman, D. (1981). *The assessment of intelligibility of dysarthric speech*. Austin, TX: Pro-ed.

Yorkston, K., Baylor, C., & Britton, D. (2017). Incorporating the principles of self-management into treatment of dysarthria associated with Parkinson's disease. *Seminars in Speech and Language*, 38(3), 210–219.

Chapter 8

Saving lost voices

A toolkit for preserving communicative identity

Jennifer Benson

Introduction

As speech and language therapists (SLTs) part of our job is to look for ways to maintain a person's communication by any means available when there is a risk that it will be lost due to disease, be that a progressive neurological condition or a cancer involving loss of, or change to, anatomical structures. Alternative and augmentative communication (AAC) is a crucial part of the SLT role within this area (see Chapter 1), and there are many high-tech voice output communication aids that can fill a gap and allow people to continue to express their thoughts, wants and wishes. But, can a generic computerised voice truly replace what has been lost – especially given the bereavement for their voice and identity that many people sense? This chapter considers this issue from a fresh perspective, that of voice banking. It first explains what voice banking and related methods entail. It then outlines issues in preparing for voice banking illustrated on the basis of someone with multiple system atrophy (MSA). And finally, it suggests a model of communicative identity.

Voice banking involves audio recording a person saying a specifically designed, standard set of phrases, which are then digitised by a commercial provider, to produce a 'synthetic' version of the person's own voice. The number of phrases required varies by provider, at present ranging from 50 to 1,600 and beyond. Once the synthetic voice is downloaded to any appropriate communication aid, it permits generation of novel utterances via direct or indirect input – that is, you can say anything in the synthetic voice in exactly the same way as you would with a generic 'voice' on a communication aid. Whilst the synthetic voice captures many aspects of an individual's original voice, it remains limited by the constraints of AAC – for example, currently, the synthetic voice lacks the subtle expression of emotion that would be found in a natural voice. At times, this may be a reason for a patient rejecting the voice or feeling that it does not reach their expectations. This underlines the importance of managing expectations of the technology from the very first discussion.

DOI: 10.4324/9781003172536-8

In **message banking** (Costello, 2016), the person chooses their own personal phrases and audio records them directly onto a computer, smartphone or other devices. The recorded phrases are then programmed into a communication aid and played back when needed. Message banking does not permit generation of novel utterances as voice banking does, and only the pre-recorded phrases will be played back on selection. On the plus side, direct recording fully captures the person's habitual voice. It is particularly suited to capturing phrases very personal to an individual, such as endearments, family names, quirky phrases, sarcasm and shared jokes. Family members and friends may play a big role in thinking of these phrases, as they can be more alert to phrases that an individual uses regularly – phrases which form a part of their communicative identity.

Video banking for some may arguably fall outside the remit of SLT, but in so far as it fits within the bigger picture of preserving communicative identity, it clearly complements voice and message banking. This tool is different as it is not always going to be used as part of an individual's communication device, although there are examples where it certainly could be. For example, a mother wishing to read a story or sing a particular song to her child may record that in a video bank. As the following case study demonstrates, the video may capture the communicative identity of an individual for use in a significant event, even after they have died, offering an added legacy element. No special equipment is needed for video banking – a smartphone or tablet is fine.

Progressive neurological conditions exemplify clearly where these interventions become critical. Motor neurone disease (MND) and MSA represent two pertinent examples. People with MND have an 80–95% chance of losing natural speech (Beukelman et al., 2011, p. 1); people with MSA have a 90% chance of the same (Miller et al., 2017). For patients who have a high probability of losing their voice because of their condition, the prospect of being able to 'keep' it can be critical to their well-being.

Voice banking also represents a potential option for some patients with head and neck cancers (Jůzová, Romportl, & Tihelka, 2015) or long-term tracheostomy. These patients may access other interventions, such as surgical voice restoration (SVR). However, these are not always suitable and involve acquiring a voice far from the person's own, original sound.

Voice banking and its siblings are relatively new tools in the SLT toolkit. As such, there is little evidence to guide practice. There remains a great need for research to answer in detail many of the questions which arise. At present, recommendations rely heavily on clinical experience and informal patient feedback. There are many works on voice banking addressing the technical and acoustic aspects of voice synthesis (not reviewed here), but few on clinical application.

Literature from the realm of voice therapy such as that by Andrews (1995) documents the psychological consequences of losing one's voice on identity and sense of self. Nathanson (2017) presents a moral case around the need for personalised voice technology to support identity and self-concept. She uses ethical principles as a theoretical framework to discuss issues around voice loss and its potential effect on an individual. Yamagishi et al. (2012) discuss technical aspects of voice banking in their chapter; however, they do also comment on the potential of voice banking application to reduce 'social distance' and maintain identity.

Cave & Bloch (2021) carried out 12 semi-structured interviews with people living with MND to examine expectations around voice banking for them and significant others. They found overall that people expressed maintenance of identity, maintenance of relationships and fighting back against the disease as reasons for banking their voices, but that expectations of how the synthetic voice was used on an AAC device, and the limitations of this were generally not well understood.

Other evidence remains anecdotal. From personal experience, patients have expressed positive attitudes to the idea and practice of voice banking. Asked whether it felt acceptable to have conversations about voice banking early in their disease course, their response has been 'yes', stressing it offered them a choice at a time when few decisions seemed to be in their hands, and it was something constructive they could focus on when everything else appeared negative. Cave & Bloch (2021) also found that 'keeping control and fighting back' was one of their overarching themes (p 125). Other patients expressed this: 'it's like an insurance policy for my voice . . . – if I don't lose it that's great, if I do lose it then I have this waiting' (Benson, 2015, p. 14). This analogy of a 'vocal insurance policy' is suggested as a way of framing what can be perceived as a difficult conversation.

Whilst there is a need for a technical provider to create the synthetic voice, the process that the SLT and client follow to complete the whole process is straightforward and easily accessible. Also, whilst the timing and content of conversations about banking can clearly be highly sensitive and emotional, SLTs experienced in working within a palliative care context and/or with long-term and life-limiting conditions will find this sits comfortably within their existing set of communication skills.

The SLT is well placed to start what may be a delicate discussion around introducing the topic of banking, having a clear and empathetic understanding of the situation the person has most likely found themselves in. They have likely received a devastating diagnosis of a disease with currently no hope of cure. They have been told that they will die, possibly within a short time. They will have learned that during that journey, they might lose their speech and many other functions. Gentle honesty helps ensure that everyone's picture of the situation and possible prognosis have been accurately and fully understood. This grows out of the more general process of educating about the particular medical condition, explaining possible prognosis and instigating longer term planning, whilst at the same time maintaining hope for the future. The possible options as regards SLT input require a similar clear and comprehensive explanation, discussion and understanding. The patient and their family need time and support to reflect on possibilities to arrive at fully informed and agreed decisions.

There are some broad service delivery issues. People who will lose their speech and voice altogether cannot wait until the disease robs them of their ability to speak before making decisions to bank or not. It needs to be whilst they can still talk. This means an SLT service must have a pathway that ensures timely referral before significant speech–voice deterioration and quick response times that allow the SLT time to work with the person and their significant others to explain and contemplate banking before it becomes too late. This typically also involves raising awareness of the benefits of voice banking with referrers to ensure that early referrals are made.

The SLT and patient do not require a detailed knowledge of voice synthesis algorithms and technology. The SLT should be able to clearly explain the advantages and disadvantages of each of the banking options, including time needed for recording. As most people are unlikely to have experience of synthetic voice, providing illustrations is vital. Ideally, the SLT has their own voice banked to present as a comparison with their live voice for the patient to evaluate. This is also useful for demonstrating the basic concept of AAC for those who may not have considered this. Experience shows this is an important step in managing expectations concerning the nature of the new voice. Fully understanding the process of voice banking by the SLT completing their own recordings is also helpful for providing support.

Personal choice around whether a synthetic voice is acceptable to an individual is a critical part of the process and can be highly personal. One person may be satisfied with a dysarthric voice that the SLT did not feel was necessarily suitable for banking; another may not accept a synthetic voice despite their family feeling it represents a good likeness. Message banking as a complementary tool can be used to bridge some of the gaps in these situations.

The concept of 'vocal insurance' is helpful here. We may not know at this point precisely how speech–voice will alter, but in the event that natural speech communication becomes problematic, having a backup voice that the person has been able to spend time producing themselves whilst they are still able can be a reassuring prospect.

As previously stated, the actual process of banking a voice is not complicated. It only requires standard computers, adequate microphone and a suitable home recording environment (e.g. free of competing ambient noise). The recording session can be conducted with breaks or over multiple sessions if the person has issues with fatigue. Review of recorded items is possible, and unsatisfactory recordings are easily re-recorded. The SLT or family member can be present to deliver prompts or other advice. Accepted phrases are automatically uploaded to the provider, who will later email the voice file for listening. At present, no purchase is necessary until the voice is downloaded to the communication aid – so if the voice is not needed or not accepted, it is not paid for.

Message banking is a less formalised process, starting with the patient and their significant others generating a list of phrases to record. As many or as few phrases as are considered important can be recorded. It may take some time to identify all the desired phrases, so it is important to start this process promptly. If the voice banking provider does not offer a message banking option alongside the voice banking, then the phrases are simply recorded item by item (each a separate file) to a chosen day-to-day device, ensuring a list of the phrases is kept for reference. When needed, the sound files are downloaded to the communication aid.

Stages for video banking: Conversations about this topic are incredibly sensitive, and the SLT must find a balance between introducing the topic in a timely manner, whilst following the lead of the patient regarding what they can tolerate thinking about. It may be useful to suggest video banking early on as an option in relation to conversations about voice and message banking but return to it later. It is critical to be guided by the agenda of the patient and be aware that different individuals handle the situation completely differently. Therapeutic relationships and trust are strengthened during the processes of voice and message banking, and this may allow the person to feel more comfortable discussing video banking further on in the journey.

Making the videos may evoke an extreme emotional reaction and may raise a number of other questions about acceptance of disease progression and death. As a clinician, ensure that you feel competent to manage this and are aware of onward referral routes for psychological support or palliative care if the patient is not already within those services. Also consider your own emotional reaction to the choice and content of the video – ensure that your own supervision and support arrangements are adequate before taking on this work.

When the patient is ready, they can decide what kind of video they wish to make – whether 'just' a simple 'Happy Birthday' rendition or more complex single or multiple speeches for specific purposes.

It is recommended to discuss whether they want to prepare a 'script' for the video or will deliver it spontaneously. Will the video be staged in a particular setting, inside or outside, what clothes represent them in that particular message and do they want 'props' (notes, a glass of champagne for a toast). It may be helpful to have a family member or friend present, but some people may also find this too upsetting, or want their recordings to remain unseen until they are used. It is also important to consider 'practice runs' before a final take.

When all feel comfortable to commence, record to the chosen device – a smartphone should give sufficient quality – and make necessary backups. Any videos for communication purposes can be downloaded to the communication aid as needed. A vital last step is to decide under what circumstances; by whom, when and where the video is to be accessed and who will know when and where to find it, especially if intended for use after the patient has died.

Case report: Jon

Jon (pseudonym), 49 years old, was diagnosed with MSA 18 months before he was first referred to the SLT. He was Icelandic and had lived in Britain for many years, developing and running a very successful business. Icelandic was his first language, which he used with family and friends. Business was conducted in English. He had a wife and two daughters and a varied social life.

Jon reported awareness of his speech changing about six months before referral to the SLT. Subjectively on first meeting Jon, his speech rate was rapid, and this affected his intelligibility; when prompted to slow down, intelligibility improved. He reported that he often had to repeat and found people looked blankly at him when they had not understood. At best, he was mildly dysarthric with slightly reduced intelligibility, but moderately dysarthric with a marked intelligibility reduction when fatigued. He reported using his Icelandic accent as an 'excuse' for how his speech sounded. Alongside his speech deterioration, Jon experienced physical changes, mainly affecting his legs, and mild cognitive difficulties, mainly around short-term memory, attention and concentration.

Jon was keen to improve his speech. Clear speech exercises were trialled focusing on slowing down and over-articulation, and strategies for pacing, but with limited success. Jon's cognitive difficulties affected his ability to maintain a slower rate or to consistently apply strategies. Jon was also very busy at work; his business was a hugely important part of his identity. Committing to therapy sessions was a low priority despite the communication challenges. Additionally, there were issues accepting the diagnosis and prognosis.

During this session, the SLT also introduced the idea of voice banking to Jon, using the framework of 'insurance for your voice'. There was a discussion of the process, how to go about it, what the finished product might sound like and how it could be used on a communication aid. The SLT demonstrated her synthetic voice as an example. It was apparent that Jon was struggling to come to terms with the changes to his life and needed to take some time to think about how life might be in the future.

Waiting at this point meant taking a calculated risk between finding acceptance of the situation and recording better voice versus waiting and risk of deteriorated voice to bank. Two weeks later, Jon contacted the SLT again, having thought about the options available and having carried out some research independently. He wished for help with the process before he lost his voice. He felt that his speech was already more difficult, though perceptually there had not been a significant change. This may have represented a further acceptance of his condition and of the likely outcome of deterioration to his speech.

The next step was to select a commercial provider to record with to produce the synthetic voice. Jon selected a provider requiring only 50 phrases to produce the synthetic voice. Finding the optimum time of day to record was critical; Jon's speech was much clearer first thing in the morning but fatigued markedly throughout the day. During recording, his self-monitoring of speech was poor, and it costs him significant effort, with ongoing prompting and cueing from the SLT, to slow down. Jon listened to recorded phrases to gain feedback on how his speech sounded. Based on this, he repeated some of the phrases to achieve his optimum voice. He completed the 50 phrases in one session at home.

Jon hated the synthetic voice that was produced. He and his wife described it as robotic, too computerised; both said it sounded nothing like him. Jon definitely did not want to hear that voice; it was too far from his own.

After discussion, Jon elected to try an alternative provider who also offered a voice repair aspect to their synthetic voice creation, which may help to compensate for dysarthria. This provider required 150–300 recorded phrases to complete their inventory. This needed more than one session, due to fatigue factors. Recording was supported by the SLT, prompting Jon to slow down and to practice a phrase prior to recording it. Items were re-recorded if necessary. Again, optimum voice for Jon was achieved through supportive, patient-focused intervention.

Jon, his wife, his friend and the SLT all agreed that the new synthetic voice provided an excellent likeness to Jon's actual voice. Importantly, Jon found it a big improvement on the previous version. Jon's wife commented that this was a voice she was happy to download to her smartphone. The importance of supporting Jon's choice here was key, in terms of both provider and timing of recording. It also exemplified how personal the perception is to an individual of what constitutes an acceptable voice.

At the same time, Jon and the SLT started to consider message banking. There were no providers offering voice banking in Icelandic, and it was important to Jon to have a way to maintain some communication in Icelandic as a huge part of his heritage, rather than just English. Over time, Jon, his family and the SLT identified personal phrases that he wished to record, aiming for phrases at the heart of Jon's communication exchanges to capture key moments. Phrases such as 'I love you', 'Daddy loves you' and 'happy birthday mate' were clear winners. Jon's wife provided phrases she felt typical of him – 'I'm just a bloody foreigner', 'I'm not just a pretty face you know' and 'I tell you something'. Some phrases were recorded in English and Icelandic, as they were identified by Jon and his wife as being ones which he would say in both languages. Jon also came up with phrases capturing his sense of humour and sarcasm: 'listen to my funny electric voice' and 'well, I am paralysed you know'. Jon's ability to communicate his sense of humour was already restricted by his dysarthria and reduced facial expression. Being able to preserve, if not enhance, these aspects of his communicative identity for future use were key. Jon commented that having these messages banked gave an added authenticity to his overall electronic communication.

Video banking

Over the time spent discussing voice and message banking, Jon began to open up more about how he was coping with MSA and how it was affecting life. Jon had two teenage daughters. During discussions, he talked about the possibility of not being alive if and when they married. He wanted to create video messages for each of them to look at on their wedding days. This was something that Jon had been thinking about for some time but had not been ready to explore. Allowing time to accept his diagnosis, to trust in the therapeutic relationship with the SLT and to appreciate the legacy aspects of the work already completed meant Jon felt ready to discuss what for him was an incredibly difficult subject.

The video was staged to represent the occasion. Jon's wife and friend were in the house and knew of his plans for video banking, but Jon was clear that it was a process he needed to complete himself with the support of the SLT, so no one would hear the speeches in advance. Jon dressed in tuxedo, with a glass of champagne to hand. Recording was an incredibly emotional experience, for both Jon and the SLT. He was frequently overcome with emotions, making it even more difficult to speak. The SLT assisted by rehearsing elements that he wanted to include, including jokes that captured his sense of humour. Jon was adamant he did not write the speeches down; he wanted them to sound as spontaneous as possible. Jon's recordings were taken on a smartphone. It feels too personal to Jon to give any further details here, but both Jon and the SLT felt that we had truly captured his personality and identity. Preserving this was important to Jon on many levels – he commented during the process that he was not afraid to die, but he was afraid of becoming paralysed. This recording of him standing upright and speaking captured his communicative identity as a strong, healthy person and a proud father. It also captured aspects of his non-verbal communication, such as his gestures and facial expressions. After many takes, Jon was happy with his recordings, ready to edit by Jon himself with some family videos to form the finished version. After the recordings, Jon and his wife, his friend and the SLT discussed the process – this served as a 'debrief' and helped to bring Jon's mood back up. The SLT was able to debrief with a colleague to reflect in particular on the emotional intensity of the experience and the undoubted privilege of witnessing something so very personal.

Jon does not yet require AAC. That will be the next stage and will depend on a number of variables, including his communicative success in different environments. Jon recently found that some evenings when he is particularly tired, his speech can be unintelligible, and the SLT encouraged him to use the voice bank provider's text to speech app in those situations, to augment his spoken communication and 'practice' using AAC.

Jon was clear on his long-term AAC needs. Discussions focused around possible hardware, software and access options, with access being a critical part of the conversation due to Jon's awareness of his changing physical needs and likelihood of being unable to use his hands to make direct selections on a communication aid. Environmental control and computer access were also part of the discussion, as they will be key to maintaining independence over some aspects of his life. He is also interested in making further videos, with a view to being able to create a synthetic voice in Icelandic in the future if that technology becomes available.

Discussion

As an SLT, this took many skills – listening, encouraging and responding to Jon's emotional state; explaining his emotional lability and separating that from his emotional response and planning, staging, counselling and reinforcing. SLTs working in a palliative care model can be used to discussions of death and dying, and this work allowed for some valuable moments for Jon. It brought up a number of issues for Jon about acceptance of his condition overall, some of which we talked about and some of which he took away for further psychological support. It strengthened our therapeutic relationship, which will undoubtedly be of enormous value in the future as Jon's condition deteriorates.

Patients living with a progressive neurological condition face many challenges which can rob them of their identity. Identity is a complex concept made up of many facets, with voice forming a critical dimension, unique to each one of us and fundamental to our sense of self. Jon's wife commented that 'this disease is making him lose his identity a piece at a time'. Jon's feeling was that the work carried out would help to preserve and maintain his identity. At the time of writing, Jon's voice change has evened out; he continues to communicate verbally, although it is more difficult when fatigued. The SLT continues to review Jon's communication ability regularly to monitor for deterioration.

Voice banking, message banking and video banking all aim to preserve communicative identity. The impact of these interventions with an individual is not yet widely studied or fully understood, but single case descriptions are powerful in demonstrating the value of the interventions and the opinions of the people who are receiving them, which can then be utilised to inform intervention and decision-making for a wider range of people.

Sometimes, there may not be time to gain extensive amounts of recorded material – voice may have deteriorated rapidly or referral to an SLT may not have been in time. If dysarthria is present when recording, the synthetic voice will sound dysarthric. However, this may still be preferable to a generic electronic voice.

If time is short, voice fatigue is an issue and voice loss is imminent, even capturing a few short messages in the person's own voice to add to their communication aid may go a long way to preserving a little of their communicative identity.

Video banking can have multiple functions in identity preservation. However, the authenticity for personal identity is balanced against daily communication usability. If time constraints occur, it may be that video banking can be used later on using the synthetic voice and message banked phrases on the communication aid, if this is acceptable to the patient. Given the emotional content of many of these messages, it may be too difficult early on after diagnosis to record the longer messages they want to say. They may need more time to prepare them. Patient choice is key. The SLT must quickly build a robust therapeutic relationship with the patient in order to facilitate these often difficult and emotional choices, alongside fulfilling the rest of the SLT role in considering more traditional speech–voice therapy options and working with communication partners to enhance skills.

The impact of communicative identity work on family and friends can also not be underestimated. The wife of a person with MND commented that her biggest fear was forgetting what her husband sounded like – she was in touch with a number of other relatives of people with MND who had mentioned that was their experience. She was also concerned about the impact on their children of never hearing their father's voice again and how that would affect their ability to cope overall with the impact of MND. This family found that continuing to hear the person they loved communicating in his own voice helped to mitigate some of the losses and that even though the voice was synthetic, it represented a great comfort to them. After his death, his wife kept the voice recordings to listen to when she was ready and that legacy of his voice remained with the family forever. She became a great advocate of voice banking and went on to promote its use more widely.

Cave & Bloch's (2021) significant others mainly commented about the benefits of voice banking on their relative with MND's identity, mood and relationships, but it is likely that there is an impact on both the person with and MND and their significant others. Indeed, Nathanson (2017, pp. 74–75) notes that 'the sound of someone's voice sets in motion a rich pattern of affective, biographical and visual experiences and memories that combine to create a sense of the speaker in the listener and contribute to the current and historical experience of that relationship'. Communication is not one sided and is always representative of a relationship, occurring within a social network or situation, influenced by intrinsic and extrinsic factors which influence the overall interaction.

Figure 8.1 proposes a model of communicative identity as a framework for discussions with patients. Communicative identity brings together a number of factors which make our individual communication unique. It is dynamic, constantly growing, evolving and changing in response to internal and external influences. With this in mind, communicative identity has been represented as a series of interrelated cogs – continually turning around the central cog. By considering as many of these aspects of communicative identity as possible in discussions with patients, the hope is to capture and preserve as much of a person's communicative identity as possible.

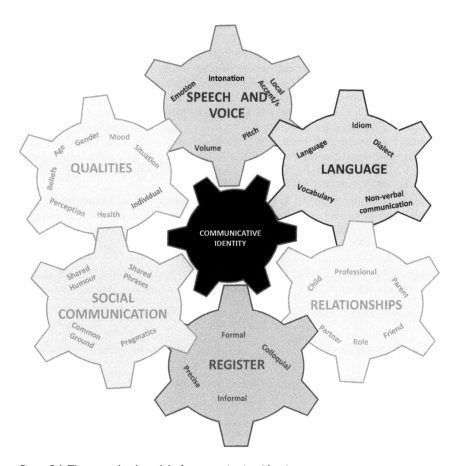

Figure 8.1 The cog-wheel model of communication identity

Returning to Jon to conclude, voice and message banking aimed to preserve the aspects of Jon's speech and voice, both his languages and vocabulary, his relationships and register and his social communication. We captured him as a proud father on video, catching those more subtle aspects including his non-verbal communication and how he perceives others to see him as a communicator. Jon's communicative identity was preserved, ready for integration into his communication aid when he is ready.

Now do you think that just providing the communication aid is enough?

References

Andrews, M. L. (1995) *Manual of voice treatment: Pediatrics through geriatrics.* Singular Publishing Group.

Benson, J. (2015) Have your MND patients taken out their vocal insurance yet? *Bulletin of the Royal College of Speech and Language Therapists*, December 5, 12–14.

Beukelman, D., Fager, S., & Nordness, A. (2011) Communication support for people with ALS. *Neurology Research International*, 2011, 714693.

Cave, R. & Bloch, S. (2021) Research report: Voice banking for people living with motor neurone disease: Views and expectations. *International Journal of Language and Communication Disorders*, January/February 56(1), 116–129.

Costello, J. (2016) *Message banking, voice banking and legacy messages*. Boston Children's Hospital. https://mymessagebanking.com/

Jůzová, M., Romportl, J., & Tihelka, D. (2015) Speech corpus preparation for voice banking of laryngectomised patients. In Král, P. & Matoušek, V. (eds.), Text, speech, and dialogue, TSD 2015: Lecture notes in computer science, vol 9302. Springer, Cham. https://doi.org/10.1007/978-3-319-24033-6_32

Miller, N., Nath, U., Noble, E., & Burn, D. (2017) Utility and accuracy of perceptual voice and speech distinctions in the diagnosis of Parkinson's disease. PSP and MSA-P *Neurodegenerative Disease Management*, 7(3), 191–203. doi:10.2217/nmt-2017-0005

Nathanson, E. (2017) Native voice, self-concept and the moral case for personalized voice technology. *Disability and Rehabilitation*, 39(1), 73–81.

Yamagishi, J., Veaux, C., King, S., & Renals, S. (2012) Speech synthesis technologies for individuals with vocal disabilities: Voice banking and reconstruction. *Acoustical Science and Technology*, 33(1), 1–5.

Chapter 9

A better conversations approach for people living with dysarthria

Steven Bloch and Suzanne Beeke

Introduction

In this chapter, we present the case of Nick and Dorothy (pseudonyms). Nick is a man with Parkinson's disease and hypokinetic dysarthria characterised by reduced volume and pitch. He also has bradykinesia (slowness of movement). Dorothy is his conversation partner (CP). This case report follows the CARE guidelines (Riley et al., 2017).

Better conversations (BC) is an intervention designed for use by speech and language therapists (SLTs) to support people with communication difficulties to have more enjoyable interactions in their everyday lives. It involves working in collaboration with these people and their regular communication partners to identify their own priorities, to promote positive conversation strategies (facilitators) and to reduce any barriers that lead to problems. The therapy itself is based on a clear understanding of each couple's existing communication profile: what they find easy in conversation as well as areas that are challenging. The key principle is that conversations are highly individual to particular speakers. One-size-fits-all strategies are not as helpful as those tailored to the conversational style of the partnership. BC also recognises that strategies need to be the focus of therapy and not just add-on suggestions at the end of a session; practice and facilitated reflection are key. The starting point for the approach is an SLT's observation of a dyad's everyday conversations using recordings (audio or video) made in as natural an environment as possible. Such observations are used as a central part of the conversation assessment and as part of feedback in the therapy.

The case presented here is unique given that it is the first published account of the BC approach for people living with Parkinson's disease and dysarthria. We focus on one specific goal (responses to a CP's turns) and show how the participants' conversation behaviours change in line with the therapy objectives.

Participant information

Nick, a 72-year-old retired security consultant, living in the south of England, was recruited to a BCD feasibility study. Ethical approval was obtained from

DOI: 10.4324/9781003172536-9

a UK National Health Service Research Ethics Committee. Full consent was obtained as part of the recruitment process. Nick had been diagnosed with Parkinson's disease by a neurologist ten years prior to the study and, at the time of recruitment, was classified as Stage 2.5 on the Hoehn and Yahr Scale (Hoehn and Yahr, 1967). There were no reported comorbidities. At the time of this study, Dorothy was a 70-year-old woman, neurotypical and having been married to Nick for 45 years.

Primary symptoms and concerns of the participants

In the previous four years, Nick's speech had been characterised by hypo-kinetic dysarthria featuring significantly reduced volume and some slowness of articulation. There was also some loss of facial expression and slowness of movement and initiation. Nick's primary concern was not being understood, particularly in group settings but increasingly at home with Dorothy. Dorothy's primary concern was a perceived lack of response from Nick when she talked to him. She was unsure whether he always understood her or not or whether he was even interested in what she had to say. Hearing and vision were unimpaired based on patient report and observation.

History

There was no reported family history of neurological disorders and no reported mental health issues. Both Nick and Dorothy reported strong local community support through participation in the church and as active followers of a local football team. They had three adult children and four grandchildren.

Relevant past speech and language therapy interventions with outcomes

Within the three years prior to the BCD treatment, Nick had engaged with one-to-one Lee Silverman Voice Treatment – LSVT® (Ramig et al., 2018) and also more general communication support in a local speech and language therapy group. He reported reasonable satisfaction with LSVT® but found the intensity and regularity of the sessions difficult. He felt that his voice was louder during therapy but did not feel that this had generalised to everyday life. He found the group work enjoyable but did not feel it made a significant difference to his overall communication. Dorothy reported that the communication support group was helpful for her in terms of meeting other partners/carers. She felt that the LSVT® had been a considerable amount of work for Nick and had led to some fatigue.

Clinical findings

Assessment: pre-therapy assessment

Nick's speech was classified by the first author as demonstrating moderate-to-severe hypokinetic dysarthria. He was difficult to understand in conversation. Intelligibility was measured using the Assessment of Intelligibility of Dysarthric Speech (Yorkston, Beukelman, and Traynor, 1984). The results revealed 40% intelligibility for single words and 63% intelligibility for sentences.

A conversation baseline measure was taken: a video recording of the dyad engaged in conversation at home. The dyad (Nick and Dorothy) was asked to talk about their day-to-day plans and activities with no preset conversation topics. The SLT set up a standard digital camera on a tripod, started the recording and then left the room, returning to turn the camera off. The dyad recorded themselves in conversation 30 minutes before therapy and 30 minutes after therapy.

From the recording, a number of barriers and facilitators were identified by the SLT. These are summarised in Figure 9.1.

From a pre-therapy interview, Dorothy's primary concern was a perceived lack of response from Nick when she spoke to him. Nick did not show the same level of awareness but was concerned about the potential impact of his communication problems on Dorothy. A review of the pre-therapy video

	Nick	Dorothy
Facilitators	• Allows time for Dorothy to talk • Orients to Dorothy well • Ability to take next turn when given time	• News worthiness of topics • Copes well with quiet speech • Comments positively on what Nick says • Allows Nick time to respond • Looks to Nick near end of turns
Barriers	• Minimal turns • Slow response • Reduced facial expression	• New topic initiation too frequent? • Doesn't often ask direct questions to elicit a response

Figure 9.1 Barriers and facilitators

01	D:	lucky that they've asked us really, I think it's lovely that
02		they've asked us (gazes to Nick)
03	→	(1.5 second silence)
04		for David you know, not his parents (gazes to Nick)
05	→	(5.5 second silence)
06		be lovely to be with the girls for a week (gazes to Nick)
07	→	(4.5 second silence)
08		an hopefully in August we'll have some nice weather (gazes to Nick)
09	N:	yeah
10	D:	(*nods*)

Figure 9.2 Extract from pre-therapy conversation

did provide evidence for how Nick was responding to Dorothy. This was particularly apparent for what we call assessments or evaluations initiated by Dorothy (e.g. expressing a positive or negative opinion about someone or something). If Dorothy expressed a view about something in conversation, there was often a next turn opportunity for Nick to share his own view or stance (see Pomerantz, 1984) but what followed was often a lengthy silence. It was not the case that Nick never spoke or never gave an opinion but that he did so far less often than might be expected. This absence of responses by Nick is illustrated in Figure 9.2 (see '→' for specific turns where a next turn response might be expected).

A review of the video recording identified 13 'evaluative' instances. All 13 featured Dorothy making an evaluation or assessment that could be followed by an agreement or further evaluation/assessment by Nick. There was evidence of just three such next turns by Nick.

Post-therapy assessment

As with the pre-therapy session, a 30-minute video of the dyad in day-to-day conversation was recorded without the SLT present. This was followed by a semi-structured interview to discuss acceptability and feasibility of the therapy for the participants (see the following sections for further details).

Additional assessments

Nick and Dorothy's perspectives were elicited through weekly written feedback during the BCD intervention and also in a post-therapy interview.

Therapeutic intervention

The BCD programme comprised six direct face-to-face treatment sessions. All sessions were scheduled according to the availability of the dyad and took place in their home to maximise natural interaction. Each therapy session lasted 90 minutes and took place approximately one week apart (±two days) over a

1	Name	Better Conversations with Dysarthria
2	Rationale	To identify and increase facilitators to conversation and reduce barriers to conversation (drawing on the methods and findings of conversation analysis, and on behaviour change theory).
3	Materials	Video recording of the dyad in conversation, session plans and accompanying worksheets for recording observations and reflections on tasks carried out. See Bloch (2013) for examples.
4	Procedures	Six treatment sessions encompassing: a. Discussion of the dyad's current understanding of communication and conversation, raising awareness of conversation barriers and facilitators b. Discussion around how dysarthria can impact conversation c. Reviewing video clips of dyad's interaction taken as a baseline measure d. Ongoing reflection on understanding why identified facilitators work as they do and why identified barriers cause difficulties – include discussion on contextual factors (e.g. time of day, concurrent activities, potential emotions associated with specific topics). e. Ongoing role play with clinician to identify and reinforce positive strategies and to reduce challenges in conversation, aided by a checklist. f. Explanation re: conversation actions or sequences relevant to dyad – particularly with reference to repair (resolving problems when they occur). g. Discussion re: different ways of managing problems with unintelligibility (or other relevant features). h. Ongoing reinforcement of importance of barriers and facilitators. i. Reviewing the programme and key take home points such as the focus being on conversation and interaction and the dyad, rather than an individual. A summary of feedback on progress and performance from clinician. j. Reviewing goals discussed in previous sessions and discussing generalisation and sustainability.
5	Who provided	A research SLT with 20+ years of experience of working with adults with progressive neurological conditions in the community with a focus on participation and everyday conversation.
6	Modes of delivery	1:1 face to face (co-present)
7	Location	The dyad's own home
8	When and how much	Weekly over a six-week period, with each session lasting 90 minutes.
9	Tailoring	Session 1 was standardised but the content of the therapy in subsequent was tailored to address the specific priorities of the dyad and
10	Modifications	One modification with reference to the use of video feedback (see below)

Figure 9.3 Treatment overview based on the TIDieR (Template for Intervention Description and Replication) checklist (Hoffman et al., 2014)

six-week period. Total contact time was nine hours. The therapy sessions were delivered by the first author in the capacity of a research SLT with over 25 years' experience of direct clinical and applied research work with people with progressive neurological conditions. Therapy sessions were filmed to provide a record of the delivery and content of therapy and to support programme evaluation.

The therapy itself, summarised in Figure 9.3, was designed in collaboration with a specialist SLT advisory group and informed by ongoing applied research work on dysarthria in conversation (Bloch, 2013; Bloch and Wilkinson, 2009, 2011a, b; Griffiths et al., 2012). It was also informed by better conversations with Aphasia (Beeke et al., 2013).

Follow-up and outcomes

Here, we report two outcomes: changes in conversation behaviour as assessed through the post-therapy video and participant report outcomes as assessed through the post-therapy interview.

01	D:	I'm really pleased with that garden out there, are you?
02		(0.5)
03	N:	yeah it's a brilliant job
04	D:	mm ((nods))
05	N:	really good

Figure 9.4 Extract from post-therapy conversation

Changes to conversation behaviours

Based on the post-therapy video, we saw a marked increase in next turn uptakes from Nick, both for the specific area we targeted but also more generally. As this is based on a feasibility study, we cannot be conclusive in reporting our behaviour change outcomes, but there are indications of a clear difference between the pre-post recorded conversations with reference to how Nick responded to Dorothy.

As stated, prior to therapy, there were 13 'evaluative' instances. All 13 featured Dorothy making an evaluation or assessment that could be followed by an agreement or further evaluation/assessment by Nick. There was evidence of just three such turns by Nick.

Post-therapy, there were 12 evaluative instances. Six of these were initiated by Dorothy and six by Nick. In all six of those initiated by Dorothy, Nick followed with an agreement or further evaluation/assessment with no silence between turns lasting more than one second. See Figure 9.4.

Participant reported outcomes

Both Nick and Dorothy reported that the therapy helped them to talk about the effect dysarthria was having on them as individuals and the influence of this on their relationship. Understanding and acknowledging their difficulties together was reported to help reduce barriers for them in their relationship.

NICK: *It has not only helped us to communicate better it has increased my understanding of the effect my speech problems have on Dorothy.*
[Researcher: what's working well?]
NICK: *Knowing that Dorothy understands how difficult it is for me to respond immediately to questions.*
DOROTHY: *But it was this feeling that he was disappearing almost. That he was less affectionate. He was inside – but it just wasn't demonstrated which is what he needed to understand – why I was how I was. But I needed to understand that as well and I didn't come to terms with that until we'd spoken to the SLT . . . I just don't feel that we have any barriers any more . . . Like all these simple things they mean quite a lot when you get them going. They make a difference.*

Nick and Dorothy explicitly mentioned appreciating feedback on the positive aspects of their communication, describing it as 'encouraging' and 'needed'.

NICK: *[The SLT] asked me how I felt and I said I was shocked at my non-reaction to anything, he pointed out that I did in fact react.*

DOROTHY: *And you instigated a change in conversation where you offered a different point of view in the conversation.*

NICK: *Yes, he said I showed a reaction when people were talking – facially.*

DOROTHY: *You found that really useful didn't you. Not just useful but encouraging which you needed.*

Another outcome was one of self-awareness. With a core focus on feedback and self-reflection, we saw an increased confidence in talking about communication both in the abstract and in relation to Dorothy and Nick's own lives. It became clear that they had never had this opportunity before despite having engaged in SLT over a period of years. The impact of this awareness became evident in some unexpected problem-solving. Dorothy, for example, realised that Nick didn't necessarily have to be talking to show he was interested. This led to a self-generated solution whereby they would simply sit closer and hold hands whilst watching television, a seemingly small change that had a big impact on their communicative ease and emotional well-being.

Challenges to participation in the therapy

Dorothy and Nick noted that occasionally their engagement with the intervention was challenged:

NICK: *I was extremely tired this week and my voice was week. Communication was difficult.*

NICK: *I can't write so Dorothy had to go through my diary, which wasn't a problem.*

Adverse and unanticipated events

There was one adverse event to report. The BC approach has been developed with bespoke video feedback reflection as a key feature. This had been explained to the dyad as part of the consent and pre-therapy introduction process. Despite this, Nick's negative reaction to seeing himself on video was unexpected and something that required immediate intervention. This event did not prevent the programme from continuing but did alter the way in which the tasks were delivered. As a result of Nick's reaction, the planned video reflection task was immediately adapted within the session to focus on the SLT's own analysis of the pre-therapy recording and also extended to enable Nick and Dorothy to reflect on how they were both communicating during the session itself.

Participant perspectives

Nick and Dorothy reported that after the BCD intervention, they were better able to cope with dysarthria. They reported benefiting from time spent on next turn uptakes simple strategies as well which improved intelligibility such as a non-verbal signal, supporting comprehension with lip reading, slowing down and taking a breath. They also reported benefitting from the suggestion of a set time in the evening for non-verbal communication – when speech was most difficult.

DOROTHY: *The suggestion to sit together on the sofa at times during the day worked very well for us. The opportunity of non-verbal communication (touch, eye contact) was good and resulted in a reduction in the feelings of isolation and separateness.*

Dorothy described how spending time with Nick and the SLT together helped her to talk more openly about issues in their relationship relating to dysarthria, which they hadn't discussed before:

DOROTHY: *With other systems you could have somebody just wanting to work on your voice. We've almost took it for granted now that there's nothing that's going to improve your voice now. We've almost got used to that. But being able to cope with it means talking to each other and with dysarthria that tends to get pushed in to the background.*
DOROTHY: *It wasn't until we talked about it with [the SLT] that I put it into words and I had no idea about it. We're very good at talking to each other but we didn't manage that did we.*

Dorothy acknowledged that she had been feeling disconnected from Nick because of his reduced responses. This was described by Nick as '*a revelation*' and led to practical problem-solving for the couple. This is particularly interesting as Dorothy and Nick described their relationship as one with lots of positive communication: '*There are times when we've talked in to the night and gone to bed really late because we've just talked and talked and talked . . . We always have something to talk about don't we*'. This, along with the comment from Dorothy above '*we didn't manage that, did we*' suggests that there is a need to explore communication and to problem-solve even for couples who rate their own communication as positive and are experiencing speech difficulties which are 'mild'.

Discussion

A BC approach aims to identify and address areas that will make a difference to the everyday lives of people with communication disorders. It does this by working with participants to identify and promote facilitators that make conversation easier/more enjoyable and to reduce barriers that make conversation problematic.

Nick and Dorothy took part in a feasibility trial of BCD. The therapy approach, session plans and resources were developed to support a six-session programme. The therapy programme was designed to be flexible enough to respond to the overall needs of the participants and the moment by moment responses to the activities and ideas being presented.

The outcomes of this early work have been promising. The participants as well as the SLT found the experience rewarding and interesting. There is also evidence that a targeted approach can change the conversation behaviour of a person with Parkinson's disease.

A greater openness and knowledge around their own communication supported Nick and Dorothy to take a more reflective approach to their conversations together when faced with barriers. This is a useful outcome as the ability to reflect together on their communication is something they can continue to use to problem-solve for themselves. It also suggests the understanding that their communication is a joint responsibility. Interestingly, this dyad also felt that they benefitted from reflecting on the programme in between sessions via the feedback forms. This could suggest that reflection is applied more readily by some couples and it may be that others require support to reflect or understand how reflection could benefit them.

There were two important issues that had not been expected. The first was Nick's reaction to seeing himself on video. The BC programme had been developed with bespoke video feedback reflection as a key feature. This had been explained to the dyad as part of the consent process and in the early therapy work. Despite this Nick's negative reaction to seeing himself on video was unexpected and something that required specific intervention. The result was positive, but it was a clear indication that sensitivity is required when using video feedback. SLTs should certainly not assume this will be unproblematic even if clients agree to its use. One option is to use video clips of *other* people if available and if there is consent. The key here is to ensure that there are appropriate examples of specific communication features to share. The second issue relates to the importance of the therapeutic alliance (Elvins and Green, 2008) for the BC approach. For this case, there is little doubt that establishing and maintaining an appropriately collaborative relationship was integral to this self-reflective behaviour change programme. The SLT was not just delivering the programme but was part of the therapeutic process itself. To this end, the impact and efficacy of a BC approach needs to be understood in the context of the broader interaction between therapist and client(s). This may be more relevant than more structural/ physiological interventions.

Key messages

- Conversation involves interaction between two or more people. Enabling conversations to work better means doing therapy with *both* the person with the communication difficulty and a key communication partner.
- The better conversations approach to therapy starts with understanding how a dyad's conversation works and the dyad's own priorities for communication.
- It aims to promote strategies that help conversations flow (facilitators).
- It also aims to reduce behaviours that hinder the flow of conversation (barriers).
- Feedback and facilitated reflection are key to making change.

References

Beeke, S., Sirman, N., Beckley, F., Maxim, J., Edwards, S., Swinburn, K. and Best, W. (2013). *Better conversations with Aphasia: An e-learning resource.* Available at: https://extend.ucl.ac.uk/

Bloch, S. (2013). Conversation and interaction in degenerative diseases. In Yorkston, K. M., Miller, R. M. and Strand, E. A. (Eds.). *Management of speech and swallowing in degenerative diseases* (Third ed. pp. 195–220). Austin, Texas: Pro-Ed.

Bloch, S. and Wilkinson, R. (2009). Acquired dysarthria in conversation: Identifying sources of understandability problems. *International Journal of Language and Communication Disorders* 44(5), 769–783.

Bloch, S. and Wilkinson, R. (2011a). Acquired dysarthria in conversation: Methods of resolving understandability problems. *International Journal of Language and Communication Disorders* 46(5), 510–523.

Bloch, S. and Wilkinson, R. (2011b). Conversation analysis and acquired motor speech disorders in everyday interaction. In Lowit, A. and Kent, R. (Eds.). *Assessment of motor speech disorders* (pp. 157–174). San Diego, CA: Plural Publishing Group.

Elvins, R. and Green, J. (2008). The conceptualization and measurement of therapeutic alliance: An empirical review. *Clinical Psychology Review* 28, 1167–1187.

Griffiths, S., Barnes, R., Britten, N. and Wilkinson, R. (2012). Potential causes and consequences of overlap in talk between speakers with Parkinson's disease and their familiar conversation partners. *Seminars in Speech and Language* 33(1), 27–43.

Hoehn, M. and Yahr, M. (1967). Parkinsonism: Onset, progression and mortality. *Neurology* 17(5), 427–442.

Hoffmann, T. C., Glasziou, P. P., Boutron, I., Milne, R., Perera, R., Moher, D., Altman, D. G., Barbour, V., Macdonald, H., Johnston, M., Lamb, S. E., Dixon-Woods, M., McCulloch, P., Wyatt, J. C., Chan, A. W. and Michie, S. (2014). Better reporting of interventions: Template for Intervention Description and Replication (TIDieR) checklist and guide. *British Medical Journal* 348, g1687.

Pomerantz, A. (1984). Agreeing and disagreeing with assessments: Some features of preferred/dispreferred turn shapes. In Atkinson, J., Heritage, J., Oatley, K. (Eds.). *Structure of social action: Studies in conversation analysis* (pp. 57–101). Cambridge: Cambridge University Press.

Ramig, L., Halpern, A., Spielman, J., Fox, C. and Freeman, K. (2018). Speech treatment in Parkinson's disease: Randomized Controlled Trial (RCT). *Movement Disorders* 33(11), 1777–1791.

Riley, D. S., Barber, M. S., Kienle, G. S., Aronson, J. K., von Schoen-Angerer, T., Tugwell, P. et al. (2017 Sep). CARE 2013 explanation and elaborations: Reporting guidelines for case reports. *Journal of Clinical Epidemiology* 89, 218–235.

Yorkston, K., Beukelman, D. and Traynor, C. (1984). *Assessment of intelligibility of dysarthric speech.* Austin, TX: Pro-Ed.

Chapter 10

Concluding thoughts

Nick Miller and Margaret Walshe

A mantra of the last decades has been that large-scale, statistically highly pow-ered randomised controlled trial (RCT) evidence provides the only answer to clinical issues around whether given interventions are successful or not, and for whom, when and under what circumstances. There is an undeniable cen-tral role for such approaches. However, many have also argued that relegating case studies and case reports to the lowest levels of evidence-based medicine misses much rich evidence that can be directly gleaned and applied in a busy varied clinic outside of generously funded research institutions (Dobinson & Wren 2019; Husain 2021; Ortega-Loubon et al. 2017)

First, there is often a gap between performance elicited in experimen-tal research trial settings and a busy day-to-day clinic. Case reports play an important role in testing and elucidating the instantiation of wider evidence-based findings. Several chapters in this volume illustrate that very clearly.

Second, the strength of a single case perspective arises from the sheer vari-ability with which dysarthria manifests itself (Schowalter et al. 2021) and the huge variation in the effects it does or does not have on the person with dys-arthria and their family. Case reports permit a much more intimate examina-tion of this and how evidence-based procedures and interventions are applied to highly individual circumstances. Chapters 2–9 all provide such examples.

Third, many argue that, especially with a disorder that manifests in such a variety of ways, large-scale RCTs cannot hope to capture the individual fac-tors that come into play. A complementary approach therefore is to provide well-controlled, systematically conducted and documented therapy in the day-to-day clinic, either through case reports such as those in this book or via more experimentally designed N-of I case studies (Murray 2019). Both case studies and case reports put the patient at the very core of clinical decision-making. This has been the main rationale driving the choice of chapters for this volume. That is, for most chapters taking individuals from the general caseload of an ordinary hospital or community clinic, with all the hurdles and compromises that are present for carrying out research.

Based on these cases, we have aimed to highlight the assessment and inter-vention thought processes and dilemmas faced on a day-to-day basis. We have

DOI: 10.4324/9781003172536-10

acknowledged that things sometimes never seem to go to plan – the initial diagnosis turns out to be wrong, the initial focus of therapy transpires not to be the best and what looked like the correct intervention needs to be modified. Nevertheless, or even despite this, the chapters illustrate that it is possible to use routine clinical cases to advance our understanding of dysarthria in general, of particular differential diagnostic conundrums (Chapter 2) and to demonstrate the utility and success of specific approaches to assessment and intervention that large-scale studies have suggested should be profitable (Chapters 4, 5 and 6).

Above all, we hope this volume has shown, yet again, that our patients are our greatest asset in furthering the study of dysarthria and similar conditions. By attuning assessment, intervention and long-term perspectives to their needs and responses, it helps us to better understand not only the impact of dysarthria but also the impact of the SLT's behaviour and interventions on the individual's evolving status. This close bond delivers valuable insights into what works, how it works, for whom, when and how. But, it only does that if a rigorous, valid, reliable, systematic attitude to evaluation and intervention is applied. The cases in this text demonstrate too that such an attitude is, and should be, well within the capability of any clinician. An advanced training in research, working in a prestigious research-oriented institution, is not a prerequisite.

This book is not intended as a state-of-the-art review of evidence-based intervention for dysarthria and notwithstanding the limitations that exist with single case reports, we believe it offers some examples of how to apply state of the art findings in daily routine. It has also portrayed how to contribute to advanced knowledge through one's own systematically recorded and reflected on day-to-day work. The chapters offer neither a general recipe book nor a 'how to', 'cook book' perspective – though certainly they provide valuable insights and templates for action. Rather, they provide examples that illustrate the seemingly infinite variability in the manifestation of dysarthria, the huge range of individuals who are impacted by it and the breadth of ways in which they are affected. They also reiterate the so often emphasised injunction to adopt a holistic approach – to the individual affected and the ways in which dysarthria influences their inner and outer life; they show that changes in pronunciation constitute but a minute part of that whole picture. The detail is there in chapters to help readers understand the approaches taken and to support the key message/messages within that chapter.

We hope, too, that readers, in addition to gaining valuable insights and suggestions from the case studies themselves will also be able to derive much more by consulting the supplementary materials, which afford access to dimensions seldom available in clinical case reports.

In conclusion, as we are reminded yet again that our greatest inspiration comes from our patients, we hope that this volume allows pause for reflection and inspiration on many aspects of clinical practice in dysarthria.

References

Dobinson, C. & Wren, Y. (Eds.) (2019). *Creating practice-based evidence*. London: J&R Press.

Husain, M. (2021). Time for N-of-1 trials in clinical decision-making. *Brain*, *144*(4), 1031–1032.

Murray, J. (2019). Beyond case reports: Putting the single subject design to work. In M. Walshe & M. L. Huckabee (Eds.). *Clinical cases in Dysphagia*. Oxon: Routledge Press.

Ortega-Loubon, C., Culquichicón, C., & Correa, R. (2017). The importance of writing and publishing case reports during medical training. *Cureus*, *9*(12), e1964.

Schowalter, S., Katz, D. I., & Lin, D. J. (2021). Clinical reasoning: A 33-year-old patient with left-sided hemiparesis and anarthria. *Neurology*, *96*(3), 128–133.

Index

Note: Page numbers in *italics* indicate a figure and page numbers in **bold** indicate a table on the corresponding page.

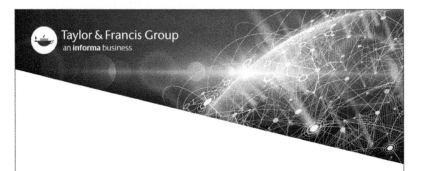

For Product Safety Concerns and Information please contact our EU
representative GPSR@taylorandfrancis.com
Taylor & Francis Verlag GmbH, Kaufingerstraße 24, 80331 München, Germany

www.ingramcontent.com/pod-product-compliance
Ingram Content Group UK Ltd.
Pitfield, Milton Keynes, MK11 3LW, UK
UKHW021455080625
459435UK00012B/517